creating a future without breast cancer

The Genesis Appeal is the UK's only breast cancer charity dedicated to the prevention of this terrible disease. It has raised funds to build Europe's first purpose-built breast cancer prevention centre, which will be opened in Manchester in 2007. The appeal is currently raising funds in order to run the centre and sponsor its staff, medical team and researchers. The hope is that this book will not only boost the appeal's funds but, even more importantly, help to get across the message that breast cancer is a largely preventable disease. For more information about the Genesis Appeal, visit *www.genesisuk.org*

We would like to express our thanks to the numerous fundraising heroes who have boosted the appeal and the many individuals, celebrity chefs and organisations who have expressed their support for this book. The following quotes are just a selection of the words of support that we have received:

'Breast cancer is an issue close to many of our hearts and one that we know is close to our members' hearts as well. Many of our leaders and members support good causes within their meetings and we actively encourage this and are proud to support such a worthy cause.

The work that Genesis undertake is unique and not only helps people on a local level in Manchester – but benefits all in looking forward to a future without breast cancer.

A number of Weight Watchers' leaders and members are of course female and that is why we are delighted to pledge our support for this book.

Our key belief at Weight Watchers is that healthy eating, physical activity and group support are key to not just losing weight, but making a massive difference in people's lives.'

WeightWatchers

'There's a saying that if diet is wrong, medicine is of no use, while if diet is right, then there would be hardly any medicine at all. The importance of eating the right foods is apparent. I welcome this book's attempt to make it so.'

Raymond Blanc

'I am very keen to support the prevention of this disease. Breast cancer affects so many people in their lifetime – men and women. I am proud to play my part in helping to spread the word about the importance of lifestyle and diet in the prevention of this terrible disease.'

Ricky Hatton
World Welterweight boxing champion

'It is with great pleasure that Wellness International and adidas support the messages promoted in this book, which represent a vital step towards the fight against cancer while at the same time helping to optimise performance and health.'

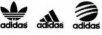

Dr Dorian Dugmore F.A.A.C.V.P.R.
Director: Wellness International at adidas

'Any sensible eating advice is valuable in helping people realise how they can eat well to maintain their health – and the consequences if they do not. It makes an important contribution to the on-going debate about diet. I also applaud the work of the Genesis Appeal – a cause of merit which deserves our support.'

Giorgio Locatelli

'Any book which stresses the importance of good diet and can also raise money to combat a disease such as breast cancer receives my warm support.'

Albert Roux

'Breast cancer affects 1 in 10 women. By buying this book you are helping support the fight against this terrible disease.'

Maureen Lipman

'It is vital that people, especially our children, realise that a good, balanced diet is essential for good health. A book like this, which helps people understand the link between the two – and on behalf of such a worthy cause – is to be appreciated.'

Brian Turner

'I have long held the opinion that healthy eating is vital to a healthy life. Indeed, Italian cuisine has become popular because it's based on wholesome ingredients that are prepared with simplicity to retain taste and nutritional value. I enthusiastically support this book.'

Pasquale Amico

'Everyone appreciates the value of good health. This book is another worthy attempt to remind people of the part they can play by eating simply and sensibly.'

Gary Rhodes

The *Genesis* Breast Cancer **Prevention Diet**

The *Genesis* Breast Cancer Prevention Diet

Dr Michelle Harvie

RODALE

This edition first published in the UK in 2006 by
Rodale International Ltd
7–10 Chandos Street
London W1G 9AD
www.rodalebooks.co.uk

Dr Michelle Harvie is a Research Dietician at South Manchester University
Hospitals NHS Trust and is sponsored by The Genesis Appeal.

adidas and the adidas logos are registered trade marks of the adidas-Salomon
AG group.

Printed and bound in the UK by CPI Bath using acid-free paper from sustainable
sources.

1 3 5 7 9 8 6 4 2

A CIP record for this book is available from the British Library

ISBN-13: 978-1-4050-9346-0
ISBN-10: 1-4050-9346-3

Notice
This book is intended as a reference volume only, not as a medical manual. The
information given here is designed to help you make informed decisions about
your health. It is not intended as a substitute for any treatment that you may
have been prescribed by your doctor. If you suspect that you have a medical
problem, we urge you to seek competent medical help. Mention of specific
companies, organisations or authorities in this book does not imply endorsement
by the publisher, nor does mention of specific companies, organisations or
authorities in the book imply that they endorse the book.

Addresses, websites and telephone numbers given in this book were accurate
at the time the book went to press.

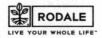

We inspire and enable people to improve their lives and the world around them

This book is dedicated to my wonderful mum Mary Harvie,
for all her love, encouragement and her amazing spirit.
Thanks for being such a great inspiration to me.

Contents

Acknowledgements

MY SPECIAL THANKS must go to Chris de Winter, who works with Genesis on project development, and who came up with the idea for this book and co-ordinated the entire project. Thanks to Alan Greene for introducing Chris to Roy Ackerman, who provided the recipes and devoted so much time and effort to overseeing their development. Special thanks to you Roy, and also to Silvena Rowe who researched the ingredients and helped develop the recipes for us. Thanks to Jenny Bowsher from Boogie Bounce, for her advice and expertise for the exercise sections of the book, John Cooper of Ikon Photography, and all our corporate supporters who have endorsed the project. Thanks also to all the celebrities and celebrity chefs who provided so much encouragement in their messages for the book, in particular Sir Trevor McDonald and Lorraine Kelly, who are patrons of The Genesis Appeal, and whose good luck messages were much appreciated.

A big thank you to the numerous women who have worked with us on the studies, without whom none of the research would be possible, and my colleagues and collaborators, including Professor Tony Howell and Professor Gareth Evans and the staff of the Breast Cancer Prevention Team at South Manchester Hospital, and Lester Barr and Genesis, for their moral and financial support for my research. Finally, thanks to my family and friends, especially Mark Garrod for his support and encouragement and for keeping me company on the hills.

Foreword

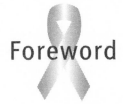

WHEN MY MOTHER DIED OF BREAST CANCER I was devastated. Our family had never known anyone with the disease and for many months before her passing we tried to pretend that she just had a bad case of flu. This was the '60s and cancer was a taboo subject in our home and many others because people had little idea of what it was or how to deal with it.

The cancer that killed my mother is a type that is easily preventable today and all women over 40 or with a history of the disease in their family should have regular mammograms and check-ups. The diagnosis and treatment of breast cancer has improved enormously since the '60s, and a smaller number of women who develop the disease die as a result of it. But sadly, as this book highlights, the number of breast cancer cases is steadily increasing. This is despite the fact that there is much that can be done to prevent this devastating disease. The majority of cases are not, as many women believe, due to genes or bad luck but to the way we live our lives, and in particular our weight and activity levels.

This is positive news because it means that there is a great deal women can do to reduce their risk of developing this unspeakable disease. And that is what this book addresses – the practical, positive steps you can take in order to avoid breast cancer. After all, prevention is so much better than cure.

Joan Collins OBE

Introduction

VIRTUALLY EVERYONE KNOWS SOMEONE, be it a relative or friend, who has had breast cancer; and the few who do not will have undoubtedly seen the newspaper headlines featuring famous women who have battled this devastating disease. Thus we hear and read about breast cancer continuously. Despite this, there is little widespread understanding amongst the public of the causes of the disease. Many people believe that their risk of developing breast cancer is largely out of their control – they will either be dealt a 'bad hand' or they will not. Whilst it is true that there are risk factors that you cannot control – for example, whether or not there is breast cancer in your family, or your age – there are also important risk factors that you can control.

The number of cases of breast cancer is increasing; 10 to 20 years ago 30,000 women were diagnosed in the UK each year, whereas now the figure is over 40,000 each year. Therein lies a clue as to how women can begin to take steps to reduce their risk of developing the disease. The rise in breast cancer cases is not due to a sudden rise in the number of people inheriting faulty genes or, as some people believe, today's more polluted atmosphere; it is a result of the way in which women's lives have changed over the recent past.

Human genes have remained much as they were thousands of years ago, but women's lives in particular have altered irrevocably. Our ancient ancestors had a large number of children early in life and breast-fed each one, were slim, ate a relatively low energy, unprocessed diet, and were highly active. Western women tend to delay having their first child, have small families, are often too busy to breast-fed, and take hormones such as the Pill and HRT. This means they have a greater exposure to the female sex hormones, which are major culprits in the development of breast cancer. No-one is suggesting women increase their family size and breast-feed in order to reduce their risk of breast cancer, but it is possible to change other features of our modern lifestyle in order to reduce the risk.

Weight and activity levels have a profound effect on breast cancer risk. On average, the amount of energy people consume (i.e. calories) has increased and the amount they expend has reduced markedly over the past few decades – to the point where 60 per cent of the population is now either overweight or obese. And as more and more studies are showing, being overweight or obese has a marked influence not only on the risk of breast cancer and indeed other cancers (womb, bowel, oesophagus) but other diseases of modern life, such as heart disease and diabetes.

None of the warnings about the risks of overweight and inactivity are new – but I believe few women realise just how much they may be able to influence their chances of avoiding breast cancer. What are the effects of losing weight, eating a healthy diet and staying fit on your risk of breast cancer? The answer from Michelle Harvie, who runs the Lifestyle programme at our Genesis Prevention Centre, is that the reduction in risk is often considerable. In this book you will find important background information concerning the latest research on breast cancer and its development, as well as all the practical information to help you make a real difference to your risk of breast cancer.

Tony Howell
Professor of Cancer Prevention
Department of Medical Oncology
Christie Hospital, Manchester

PART ONE

Understanding Breast Cancer

*'Prevention is better
than healing because it saves
the labour of being sick'*

THOMAS ADAMS, 17TH-CENTURY PHYSICIAN

The breast cancer epidemic

BREAST CANCER IS A MAJOR HEALTH CONCERN for most women. Once a taboo subject, it has been given much-needed publicity by a succession of charitable campaigns that have resulted in more and more women asking what they can do to prevent breast cancer happening to them or their loved ones. Prevention has always been a particular concern for those women with a personal family history of breast cancer – these women will most likely have experienced first-hand the pain of a loved one battling with this terrible disease – but all women need to consider the challenge that the rising incidence of breast cancer poses.

Breast cancer is the most common malignancy amongst women in the world today. Current estimates predict one in ten women in the UK, USA and Canada, and one in 11 women in Australia and New Zealand will develop breast cancer at some point in their lives. This means that each year, in the UK alone, around 40,000 women are diagnosed with breast cancer. A third of these, some 13,000 women, will die of the disease. Thankfully, the proportion of women dying from breast cancer is falling as a result of earlier diagnosis and more effective treatments. In the UK, the risk of dying from breast cancer has plummeted over the past 15 years by a staggering 30 per cent. However, while advances in treatments should be applauded, the reality of rising rates means about 1000 additional women each year, in the UK alone, have to cope with the anxiety of a cancer diagnosis and the possibility of breast surgery, chemotherapy and radiotherapy or hormone therapies. It is vital that we tackle these rising rates of breast cancer – we need to try to prevent breast cancer occurring in the first place so that fewer women have to experience the burden of this disease.

The statistics about breast cancer are alarming, but the good news is that whether or not you develop the disease is to a large extent within your own control. Contrary to what many people believe, the majority of cases of breast cancer are not due to genes or bad luck, but are hugely influenced by diet and lifestyle choices. This is borne out by the huge variations in breast cancer rates around the world (see table opposite).

In the UK one in ten women will develop breast cancer; in Australia and New Zealand the figure is one in 11 women. However, the figure for Japan is one in 35 and for India, China and East Africa it is one in 50. This means that women in the UK, Australia and New Zealand are over five times more likely to develop the disease compared to women living in India, China or some parts of Africa. These variations are not due to pre-coded differences in genetic make-up; they are the result of differences in the way we live our lives. Dramatic increases in risk are seen when Chinese and Japanese women migrate to the USA and adopt a Western lifestyle.[1]

There are many differences between the ways women live in the West compared to how women live in low risk countries, which can account for the different rates of breast cancer. The most likely 'cancer promoting' aspects of a Western lifestyle include higher weights, and the consumption of fattening, high energy, high fat, high sugar diets and lack of exercise, as well as the tendency to have fewer children, and to have children later in life (all factors that will be examined in greater detail). Earlier suggestions that a large quantity of soya in the traditional Asian diet plays a preventive role against breast cancer is not supported by recent research (see page 113). Although it is true that adopting an 'Eastern' lifestyle would probably reduce breast cancer risk, sadly, as nations such as China, Japan and India become more economically successful their populations are abandoning their traditional, healthier lifestyles and adopting more harmful Western ways. The result is that rates of the so-called 'diseases

International differences in rates of breast cancer

Country	Rates of breast cancer
UK, USA, Canada, Switzerland, Argentina, Uruguay	1 in 10
Australia, New Zealand, Italy, Denmark, Sweden, Iceland, Finland, Spain, France	1 in 11
Eastern Europe, Philippines, Saudi Arabia, Singapore	1 in 17
Northern Africa, South Africa, Brazil	1 in 25
Japan, Ethiopia, Angola, Columbia, Venezuela	1 in 35
China, India, East Africa	1 in 50

of the rich', such as heart disease and cancer, are escalating, particularly in the urbanised areas of such countries. We are seeing the greatest increases of breast cancer rates in these countries, where numbers are increasing by 5 per cent per year, compared with a 1 per cent increase in the West.

No one is advocating that women in the West should have lots of children, and have them early in life, simply to reduce their risk of breast cancer. There is a much simpler – and more effective – means of risk management available to everyone. The latest, most up-to-date research shows that controlling your weight and making wise diet and exercise choices at different stages in your life can dramatically reduce your chances of developing the disease, or of it recurring if you have already had breast cancer.

Many people are confused and sceptical about just how much effect a healthy diet and lifestyle can have on cancer risk. This is understandable given the numerous conflicting and often inflammatory stories that regularly hit the headlines. Frequently they offer false hope that eating this special food or that dietary supplement will protect us all from cancer. But of course this simply is not the case.

The greatest contribution you can make towards staying well and avoiding breast cancer, or reducing risk of recurrence for women who have already been diagnosed with the disease, is by eating a good diet, avoiding being overweight, getting an adequate amount of exercise and generally having a healthy lifestyle. With this in mind, this book gives you the facts about breast cancer, who gets it and why, and the effects of diet and lifestyle on future risk amongst breast cancer patients. You will find information on topics such as breast cancer susceptibility genes, hormones and hormone replacement therapy, but because the latest research findings closely link body weight – and hence exercise and diet – to breast cancer, these are the main areas that will be examined.

Breast cancer can begin to develop many years before it is detected. What you eat, how much you exercise and, above all, how much you weigh throughout childhood and adult life impacts on your risk. While there is nothing you can do to change what happened in your childhood, you can begin to change your diet now – and, if you have children of your own, you can give them the best start

Breast cancer in men

Men have breast tissue, but breast cancer is extremely rare in men, accounting for less than 1 per cent of all male cancers. Only 300 men develop breast cancer in the UK each year, compared to around 40,000 women. On average most of the men with breast cancer are diagnosed in their early 70s. Some male breast cancer is thought to be due to the presence of an inherited fault in genetic make-up (BRCA2 gene mutation) (see page 34). As breast cancer is such a rare condition in men it is difficult to gather good data of how to prevent the condition. However, there is some evidence that weight control and exercise may also be protective factors for male breast cancer.

in life by ensuring they eat healthily, get plenty of exercise and control their weight.

Weight control is a major challenge for many people. Everyone is so busy, fitting in looking after the family, the home and a hectic work schedule as well. It is hard to find the time to look after yourself and your own health. All these pressures make it harder to maintain a healthy weight, which adds to levels of stress. Stress is undoubtedly bad for the health too, albeit not directly linked with risk of breast cancer. Losing weight and exercising are great ways to relieve stress, and make you feel better, more empowered and more positive. There are no guarantees as to whether or not you get breast cancer, but you can work at lowering your risk by making sensible lifestyle choices. This book will help you make those choices.

Summary

- *One in ten women in the UK will develop breast cancer at some point in their lives.*

- *Women in the UK are five times as likely to develop the disease compared to women living in India or China, or some parts of Africa.*

- *Rates of breast cancer are increasing worldwide. The rapid increase in rates of breast cancer in countries such as China and Japan is due to the adoption of Western lifestyles.*

What is breast cancer?

BREAST CANCER can take a number of years to develop. Events in childhood and adolescence, such as how quickly and how much you grow, and the age that you start your periods can influence whether you go on to develop breast cancer later in life. Evidence from women who survived the atomic bomb at Hiroshima in Japan showed that it often took 20 years between the initial radiation damage and the detection of cancer.

Before going on to look at how breast cancer develops, it will be useful to examine the development of the breast.

The development of the breast

The breast begins to develop during puberty. Typically, five to ten milk ducts within each breast (which arise in the developing baby in the middle stages of pregnancy) begin to extend and branch. Each duct starts in the nipple and has many branches in the breast, which end in glands called lobules, and is surrounded by fibrous and fatty tissues, which make up the rest of the breast. Ducts and lobules are made up of small building blocks or cells, which constantly die and regenerate, depending on hormone levels. Many women are more than aware of breast swelling and tenderness in the two weeks before a period. You will not be surprised that the higher levels of hormones (oestrogen and progesterone) in the body in these two weeks leads to an increase in the activity of cells in the ducts and lobules within the breast.

The development of breast cancer

Three key steps need to occur before a tumour develops fully and is detectable. Each of these steps is potentially reversible and is known to be influenced by lifestyle, which provides numerous opportunities to interrupt the development of breast cancer. The fourth step is when the cancer spreads beyond the original site.

Step 1 Initiation

Breast cancer often arises in one of the cells lining the milk ducts or lobules in the breast, most commonly at the neck of the lobules. The genetic material in the cell becomes damaged by unstable reactive molecules in the body, or agents present in the environment, such as chemicals or radiation, or as a direct result of high hormone levels in the body that cause the cell to divide, which is a risk period for damage to the cell.

Breast cells (as with all cells in the body) are normally programmed to die and to be replaced. The damaged cell switches off these restraints, divides and does not die; the cell becomes out of control. These are the first steps of cancer development. Diet can influence these first steps. Free radicals are a by-product of any food digested and processed in the body. Inevitably production of these free radicals (and damage to cells) is highest when too many calories are consumed, especially in diets high in animal fats and alcohol. On the other hand, a good supply of protective antioxidant nutrients (vitamin C, vitamin E, beta-carotene, selenium and other chemicals found particularly in brassica vegetables, grapes and green tea) will mop up these cancer causing reactive molecules, while foods rich in folic acid can help protect your genetic material from damage (see page 111).

Step 2 Promotion

In the second key step, the damaged cell continues to multiply and make lots of copies of itself with no braking mechanism. These cells are direct copies so they all contain the same damaged genetic material, in the same way as a mistake on a sheet of paper will appear on all the photocopies made from it. Multiplication of cancer cells is driven by high levels of hormones such as oestrogen, progesterone and insulin or the presence of a long-standing, low-grade inflammation in the body. These cancer promoting factors are significantly raised in women with the highest calorie intakes, the highest weights and the most sedentary behaviour.

Step 3 Progression
If the tumour is to survive and develop further it must develop its own local blood supply. Failure to do so will mean that the tumour won't receive enough oxygen and nutrients and will starve. A tumour that does secure a blood supply and continues to grow now becomes detectable. The body naturally produces a hormone that helps block this happening; this cancer-protective hormone is lowest in the heaviest, most sedentary women, which again places them at higher risk of cancer spreading.

Key nutrients that help block a cancer's ability to develop its own blood supply are found in dairy products, fruits, vegetables and pulses and the spice turmeric.

Diet, lifestyle and cancer development

Diet/lifestyle factor	Initiation of cancer	Growth of cancer	Spread of cancer
Too many calories	▲	▲	▲
High body weight	▲	▲	▲
Lack of exercise	●	▲	▲
Fruit and vegetables	▼	●	▼
Folic acid	▼	●	●
Soya	▼ or ▲	▼ or ▲	●
Alcohol	▲	▲	●
Dairy products	●	▼	▼

Key: ▲ promotes stage of cancer development; ▼ helps to block stage of cancer development; ● no effect on stage of cancer

Step 4 Spread of cancer

Cancer cells can migrate into nearby lymph (fluid that bathes the tissues of the body) channels and blood vessels, and spread to other parts of the body, such as the bones, liver, lungs and brain. This process is known as metastasis. Cancer cells can continue to multiply and grow at sites distant from the breast, causing damage to these vital organs and, ultimately, death.

Early detection and screening
Be breast aware

All women should be breast aware. If breast cancer does arise, finding it in its early stages means there is an excellent chance of successful treatment. Put simply, early detection saves lives.

Some experts are against the practice of self-examination, believing that it leads to a lot of unnecessary worry, and indeed a series of large randomised trials found that breast self-examination (BSE) may increase the chances of unnecessary breast biopsies for benign lumps.[2] It is therefore prudent to be breast aware but bear in mind that the great majority of breast lumps will be benign.

You should look at your breasts so you know what is normal for you. Signs to look for are:
• changes in size or shape of your breasts
• dimpling on the skin of the breast
• changes in the position of the nipple (in-growing), a rash or nipple discharge
• pain or discomfort that is new, especially if it is only felt on one side (though this is rarely a sign of cancer).

These can all be signs of breast cancer but more often they are not. The likelihood of these symptoms being breast cancer is, however, higher in post-menopausal women. If you do find anything unusual, report it to your doctor without delay.

Breast screening

Breast screening does not prevent cancer but can detect it at an early stage when it is too small to be felt by either the woman herself or by a doctor. Screening involves taking X-rays of the breast in a procedure known as a mammogram. In the UK women between the ages of 50 and 70 are invited for screening every three years. Women in Australia and New Zealand are offered screening every two years. In Australia this can include women from the age of 40 upwards at their request, while women over 45 are invited in New Zealand. The benefits or otherwise of screening have been the subject of much-publicised debate. Experts agree that women should attend breast screening where it is available. The World Health Organisation's International Agency for Research on Cancer (IARC) concluded that breast screening saves lives. Women aged 50 to 69 years old attending breast screenings were 35 per cent less likely to die from breast cancer; for every 500 women screened, one life will be saved.[3] The benefits for younger women are not as clear, partly because the density of breast tissue makes it more difficult to detect problems. Women concerned that the radiation from X-rays may actually increase their chance of getting breast cancer can be reassured that the dose for each mammogram is about the same as you would routinely experience from 40 days of normal background radiation on earth!

What about breast pain?
Many women suffer from breast pain, especially in the two weeks before a period. This does not increase their risk of breast cancer. Women with severe symptoms will often be referred to a breast specialist, who may advise suitable pain relief or occasionally drugs, which lower or block the effects of the hormone oestrogen.

Summary

- *Breast cancer develops over many years and goes through three major stages of development before it is detected.*
- *Sensible diet and lifestyle choices at any of these stages can reverse any of these stages and stop cancer developing or progressing.*
- *Women should be breast aware and attend breast screening wherever it is available; early detection saves lives.*

3

'Can I influence my risk of breast cancer?'

A numbers game

The risk of getting breast cancer is described in terms of the numbers of women in a population who will develop the disease. For Western women, the risk is fairly high (see page 20) and breast cancer is unfortunately a fairly common occurrence. Your lifetime risk of developing breast cancer is far greater than, for example, the chances of getting flu each year, which is estimated to be only one in 500.

Whether you get breast cancer or not is not simply due to chance or bad luck – you can work at lowering your risk by making sensible lifestyle choices. There are of course no certainties in life. Taking the steps suggested in this book will help reduce your risk, but cannot guarantee that you will not develop the disease.

Genes versus lifestyle

Two common misconceptions are that most breast cancer is down to genetic make-up and that inheriting a faulty gene means a woman will get breast cancer regardless of the way she lives her life. As many as eight out of ten women diagnosed with breast cancer are the first to be diagnosed within their families – so breast cancer does not just 'run in families'. Only 5 per cent of cases of breast cancer are caused by strong, currently identifiable genetic factors, with a possible further 20 per cent due to yet undiscovered genes, which make women more susceptible to the cancer causing effects of lifestyle. These figures are deduced from large twin and population studies headed by Professor Julian Peto at the Institute of Cancer Research in Surrey, England,[4,5] and are consistently found in populations studied; for example only 235 of the 4730 cases of breast cancer (5 per cent) studied by researchers at Yale University School of Medicine occurred in women carrying an identifiable inherited faulty gene[6] and only 172 of the 2389 cases of breast cancer (7 per cent) within a large population of nurses studied at Harvard School of Public Health arose in women with a strong family history.[7] This means that almost 95 per cent of breast cancer results from exposure to risk factors such as weight gain, poor diet, lack of exercise, having children or not, use of the contraceptive pill or hormone replacement therapy. The huge role played by lifestyle in breast cancer risk is important news for women and their doctors, and means it may be possible to significantly reduce rates by the correct diet and lifestyle choices.

Age and breast cancer risk

Breast cancer has been known to occur in girls as young as 14 years of age. Fortunately these are rare occurrences; a woman's risk increases as she gets older. In the UK, 80 per cent of breast cancer occurs in women aged 50 years or over; most commonly between the ages of 65 and 70 years.

Breast cancer is very rare among women in their 20s and 30s. Cancers that develop at these younger ages are more likely to be due to a fault in genetic make-up and have little to do with lifestyle. This probably accounts for the apparent paradox of why breast cancer sometimes occurs in high profile, slim women leading healthy lifestyles, such as Kylie Minogue. However, many women with a family history of the disease can develop breast cancer later in life; recent research from the University of Cambridge found over half of women with a family history diagnosed with breast cancer were diagnosed some time after the menopause.[8]

Diet and lifestyle have their greatest impact on breast cancer that develops in women past the age of 35. Interestingly, rates of cancer around the world (which are known to be down to lifestyle) do not

Age and breast cancer risk

Age	Cumulative risk
Up to 25	1 in 15,000
Up to 30	1 in 1900
Up to 40	1 in 200
Up to 50	1 in 50
Up to 60	1 in 23
Up to 70	1 in 15
Up to 80	1 in 11
Up to 85	1 in 10

differ in younger women but become more obvious in women past the age of 35. A 2005 overview published in *The Lancet* attributed one in three of all breast cancer cases in women aged 40 to 70 to excess weight, lack of exercise and excess alcohol intake. The fact that breast cancer is more likely to develop later rather than earlier in a women's life, and that we stand the best chance of preventing this type of cancer with sensible lifestyle choices will be a relief to many women. Women should not however ignore their risk and put off sensible lifestyle choices until later in life. As mentioned previously, breast cancer may start to develop 20 to 30 years before it is detected. Many women in their 30s are already likely to have pre-cancerous growths within the breast. Striking evidence of this came from Danish researcher Maya Nielsen back in the late 1970s, who unexpectedly found pre-cancerous growths in one out of 12 women in their 30s and one out of three women in their 40s. These lesions would not lead to imminently detectable cancer. In fact, given the right conditions, these lesions would probably regress, while unfavourable conditions could mean these go on to develop into full-blown breast cancer in later years.[9]

The best hope of preventing breast cancer is to make sensible lifestyle choices throughout adult life. For your children and grandchildren, healthy lifestyle choices from the outset will yield the best protection against this terrible disease.

Family history and genes
Breast cancer genes and gene testing

Advances in mapping the human genome mean we will ultimately be able to identify women who are particularly susceptible to breast cancer. These women could be targeted and advised on lifestyle choices to reduce their likelihood of developing the disease. The current status of our knowledge of breast cancer susceptibility genes is however quite limited. The most well-known breast cancer susceptibility genes are the BRCA1 (BReast CAncer 1) and BRCA2 (BReast CAncer 2) genes identified in the mid 1990s. We all have these genes; their role is to help prevent cancer by making proteins that stop cells from growing abnormally and also repairing cells when things go wrong or develop faults. Mutations in these genes can be thought of as 'spelling mistakes', and may be inherited from either the mother's or the father's side. These mean that the cancer preventing protein is not as effective, putting that person at a much higher risk. BRCA1 and BRCA2 mutations increase the risk of other cancers developing in both men and women.

BRCA1 mutation genes are linked to both ovarian and colon cancer in women, and to prostate and colon cancer in males. BRCA2 mutations are linked to ovarian and pancreatic cancer in women, and to breast, prostate and pancreatic cancer in males. Mutations in BRCA1 and BRCA2 are relatively rare, occurring in 2 in 1000 women within Western populations, but in 25 in 1000 Ashkenazi Jewish women. The faulty BRCA2 gene is more common among women in Iceland, occurring in 6 in 1000 women. The relatively large numbers of Jewish and Icelandic people with faulty genes is a result of a faulty gene in one of the founder members of these populations and the fact that these populations have been established by a small number of people.

People assume gene testing simply involves a blood sample and a simple laboratory analysis. Gene testing is actually an expensive, labour-intensive process. For an analogy of the process of gene testing, imagine being given a book in a foreign language that you do not speak that is several thousand words long. You are then asked to look for a single spelling mistake in it. The only way you can find the spelling mistake is if you are given another copy of the book, which does not have any spelling mistakes, and by comparing the good copy with the faulty copy, you should eventually be able to work out the spelling mistake. You can see that this is a painstaking task!

For any particular family, the 'spelling mistake' can lie anywhere along the gene, but the same spelling mistake will be found in every affected family member. The gene fault can therefore be found by comparing the gene sequence in family members who have had breast cancer with those who have not. Once the spelling mistake for a particular family has been identified, testing other family members becomes much easier – because you now know exactly what spelling mistake you are looking for. The common 'spelling mistakes' are already known for women in Iceland or in the Ashkenazi Jewish population. Gene testing within these groups is therefore often much easier.

The scarcity of these genes, combined with the complexity of the analysis, means faulty genes are only looked for in families considered to be likely gene carriers. The biggest clue to the likely presence of these faulty genes is to have at least four close relatives who have had breast or ovarian cancer, for example, mother, daughter and sisters, particularly if they developed breast or ovarian cancer at a young age, or if men as well as women have had breast cancer in the family.

What can be done to reduce risk among known BRCA1 and BRCA2 carriers?

Inheriting either the faulty BRCA1 or BRCA2 genes does not mean that breast cancer is inevitable. Since these are faults in the genes that normally repair damage to the cells some damage must occur within the susceptible breast tissue for the cancer to develop. Nevertheless an estimated 60 to 85 per cent of BRCA1 and BRCA2 gene carriers will develop breast cancer at some time in their lives. The majority of breast cancer attributable to BRCA genes occurs between the ages of 35 and 55. Some women have their healthy breasts removed to reduce risk. The female sex hormone oestrogen is known to initiate and promote the growth of breast cancer. That is why some women opt to have their ovaries removed, which lowers levels of oestrogen and halves their risk, or alternatively to use drug therapies to lower oestrogen levels.

Careful archiving of medical records of gene carriers over the past century shows women born today with a BRCA gene fault are much more likely to develop breast cancer compared to women born with these faults more than 70 years ago. This gives the strongest indication that lifestyle can influence the susceptibility of BRCA gene carriers to developing breast cancer.

Lifestyle factors that limit gene damage and halt the progress of damaged cells are likely to be the key to preventing breast cancer among BRCA carriers. Lifestyle choices that reduce levels of oestrogen or reduce production of reactive oxidising molecules (free radicals), or alternatively increasing antioxidants that mop up these damaging molecules, may yet prove to be beneficial among BRCA carriers. A recent study from the University of Washington in Seattle, USA showed that being a healthier weight and taking regular exercise, particularly during adolescence and early adulthood, postponed the development of breast cancer in BRCA1 and 2 gene carriers by some ten years in some and prevented development in others.[10] Current research is examining whether the antioxidant selenium may benefit women with the BRCA1 susceptibility gene.[11]

Other women with a family history of breast cancer

Most women with a family history of breast cancer will not have either of the known identifiable breast cancer susceptibility genes. Such a woman is, however, likely to have as yet unidentified differences in her genetic make-up that runs in her family and influences how her body reacts to any potential cancer causing factors to which she may be exposed. Lifestyle clearly has effects on risk amongst women with a family history, which makes lifestyle choices for these women extremely important. There is even some evidence that lifestyle has a stronger effect on risk in women with a family history compared to women without. A study from the Mayo Clinic in the USA suggested that excess weight around the middle might be a particular cancer risk for women with a family history,[12] while a study from the Harvard School of Public Health in Boston, USA, showed that the consumption of fruit and vegetables was more protective against breast cancer for women with a family history.[13]

Hormonal and reproductive factors and breast cancer risk
Female sex hormones

The female sex hormones oestrogen, progesterone and prolactin are important for the normal development, growth and function (lactation) of the breast, but they are also the major culprits in stimulating the development, growth and spread of breast cancer. The more a woman is exposed to these hormones the higher her overall risk of breast cancer. Before the menopause oestrogen and progesterone are produced mainly by the ovaries. The breast is exposed to particularly high levels of both hormones during the second half of each menstrual cycle. The earlier a girl starts her periods, and the later she enters the menopause, not having children and not breast-feeding means her breasts will be exposed to a greater number of hormonal cycles and hence greater breast cancer risk. Western women today are estimated to have three times as many menstrual cycles as women who currently live a traditional hunter-gatherer lifestyle as their ancestors did 10,000 years ago[14] (see table on page 38), and thus they have perhaps 60 times the breast cancer risk.

After the menopause oestrogen is no longer produced by the ovaries but comes mainly from within the fat cells of the body by means of a specific enzyme known as aromatase. This enzyme converts some of the circulating male hormones (such as testosterone) in the blood to oestrogen. More fat means more hormone is produced. Typically after the menopause women who are 2 to 3 stone (12.7 to 19 kilograms) overweight have twice the level of oestradiol (the major component of oestrogen) in their blood than normal weight women.[15] Heavier premenopaual women can also have higher circulating levels of oestradiol, though this relationship is not as consistent as that seen in post-menopausal women. Higher levels of

Hunter-gatherer versus Western lifestyle

	Hunter-gatherer woman (Papua New Guinea)	Western woman
Age starting periods	16 years	12½ years
Age of first birth	19½	26½
Time from first period to first birth	3½ years	14 years
Number of children	6	1.8
Total time spent breast-feeding	3 years	3 months
Age of menopause	47 years	50½ years
Estimated number of menstrual cycles	160	450

oestrogen are found in women (both pre and post-menopausal) who do not exercise and who follow low fibre diets. You might wonder how fibre can be linked to blood hormone levels. This is because excess oestrogen in the body is eliminated in the bowel. Having a low fibre diet and the sluggish digestion that goes with such a diet means you will not have a healthy balance of bacteria in your bowel so oestrogen tends to be reabsorbed. With a high fibre diet and regular bowels oestrogen is less likely to be reabsorbed so it is removed more effectively from the body.

Too much oestrogen is bad news for breast cancer risk, but a complicating factor is that oestrogen is processed in the body in two different ways, to yield either a less potent form (the so-called 2-hydroxysterone form) or the more potent cancer promoting form (the 16-hydroxysterone form) in the body. As you might expect women with higher levels of the potent form and less of the less potent form are at higher risk of breast cancer. Research has shown that a potential way to promote the production of the less potent form of oestrogen is to ensure a high intake of an important nutrient found in brassica vegetables, such as broccoli, cabbage and cauliflower, known as indole-3-carbinol (see page 87).

Testosterone

You may be surprised to learn that testosterone is linked to breast cancer, or even that it is present at all in women, since it is usually considered to be a male hormone. Testosterone is made by both men and women in the adrenal gland and is naturally present in women's bodies, although at much lower levels than in men. Levels tend to be higher among heavier women, and this may be another factor that places heavier women at increased risk.

Hormone tablets

Hormone tablets containing oestrogen and progesterone, such as the contraceptive pill and hormone replacement therapy (HRT), both increase the risk of developing cancer. The additional risk of these pills is only during the time they are taken and fortunately disappears within ten years of stopping the contraceptive pill, and within five to ten years of stopping HRT.

The contraceptive pill

The best data on risk attached to taking oral contraceptives (OC) comes from an overview of 150,000 women taking OC overseen by an international collaborative group of breast cancer experts led by Professor Valerie Beral in Oxford. On average, the risk of developing breast cancer was 9 to 24 per cent higher between starting use and ten years of stopping the Pill. Since breast cancer in younger women is uncommon the actual increased risk of women taking the Pill developing breast cancer is extremely small. For example, in this population only seven additional cancers occurred in women who took the Pill between the ages of 16 and 19; 22 in women who took the Pill between 20 and 24; and 70 in women who took the Pill between the ages of 25 and 29. The effects of progesterone-only contraceptives on breast cancer risk are not known as there were too few data to analyse.

Hormone replacement therapy (HRT)

The main reason for taking HRT is to reduce the symptoms of the menopause including hot flushes, night sweats and vaginal dryness.

Breast cancer: a modern disease?

Around 100,000 years ago our genetic make-up evolved to help our ancestors endure extremely active lives. However, human genes have not changed much over the past 10,000 years or so. Many scientists believe we are still designed for a hunter-gatherer lifestyle and that many modern-day diseases such as cancer, diabetes and heart disease are the result of a mismatch between the genes inherited from our hunter-gather ancestors and the way we live now.

The chart below outlines some of the main differences.

	Hunter-gatherer 50,000–10,000 BC	21st-century woman
Pattern of eating	Spells of feast and famine	Food is constantly available – on average we eat 6 times a day
Exercise	Walk/run 5–10 miles 3–4 days per week, hunting and gathering food	Drive to supermarket/ internet shopping; 70% in the UK take less than 30 minutes' exercise per week
Fats	Plenty of lean meat, fish, nuts	High animal and saturated fat diets, i.e. fatty meat, high fat dairy, processed and baked food
Fibre	Plenty of whole grains, nuts, berries 40–50 g fibre per day	Processed white starchy foods, i.e. bread, biscuits, cake 15 g fibre per day

Oestrogen is the hormone in HRT that helps with these symptoms. For women who have not had a hysterectomy, oestrogen is combined with the other female hormone progesterone (combined HRT) to help protect the womb against developing cancer. If women have had a hysterectomy (their womb removed), oestrogen is used on its own (oestrogen-only HRT).

Two recent, highly important trials give us an indication of the degree of increase of breast cancer associated with the use of HRT. One of them, the Women's Health Initiative (WHI) study from the USA is the most important since it is the first trial (ever!) where HRT was compared with a dummy tablet in a large number of healthy women.[16] Another important trial is the Million Women Study where HRT use was followed in one million women from the national breast screening programme in the UK.[17] These studies have raised the profile in the media of the effects of HRT on health and have changed the way people think about HRT. It is important in the context of this book to look at some of the details of these investigations in more depth, as follows:

- HRT increases the risk of breast cancer.
- Combined (oestrogen and progesterone) HRT is the major culprit. The increase in the risk of breast cancer with oestrogen-only HRT is likely to be very small; oestrogen-only HRT may even reduce the risk. This may seem very surprising, but the pills use extracts of several types of oestrogen, some of which behave differently to normal oestrogen, and can actually block the effects of natural oestrogen circulating in the body.
- Risk is higher the longer combined (oestrogen and progesterone) HRT is taken.
- The increase in risk begins about one to two years after starting treatment and gradually increases further.
- Taking combined HRT in the long term (10 to 15 years) may double the risk of breast cancer during the years it is taken.
- The increased risk of breast cancer disappears within about five to ten years of stopping taking combined HRT.

The WHI study also examined the effects of combined and oestrogen-only HRT on risk of heart disease, osteoporosis and bowel cancer. Combined HRT increased risk of heart disease (25 per cent increase) and blood clots (120 per cent increase), but protected women from bowel cancer (30 per cent reduction). Both types of HRT improved bone health (30 to 40 per cent decrease in

Effect of HRT on the health of post-menopausal women

	No. of cases of various conditions per 1000 non-HRT users	Extra number of cases in 1000 HRT users	
		Oestrogen only	Combined
		5 years	5 years
Breast cancer	16	3	4
Endometrial cancer	5	4	0
Stroke	16	6	6
Clots in legs or lungs	10	5	13
Bowel cancer	7	0	-3
Fracture of hip	15	-4	-4

osteoporosis), but increased risk of stroke (40 to 50 per cent increase). The additional cases of breast cancer and other diseases among users of HRT is shown above.

The decision whether or not to take HRT is not a straightforward one. There are some other, non-hormonal agents that can help control menopausal symptoms, but HRT remains by far the most effective treatment for women with severe symptoms. Each woman needs to weigh up which of the potential benefits and risks are most important to them. If you develop mild menopausal symptoms you may prefer not to take anything after balancing up the risks and benefits, or you may wish to try one of the varieties of herbal remedies such as flax (see page 143). For women who have had a hysterectomy, their doctors might consider oestrogen-only HRT to help their symptoms, particularly, for instance, if they have had an early menopause. For women who suffer severe, intolerable menopausal symptoms the decision is maybe easier. For these women the symptoms are only likely to be helped by taking HRT. Should this be the case, it makes sense that the treatment is only taken for a couple of years or at least for as short a period as possible.

Many breast cancer patients suffer with hot flushes and, if you are one of these, you should exert caution with certain natural supplements. Options for breast cancer patients to manage menopausal symptoms are covered in detail on page 143.

The effects of pregnancy and breast-feeding

Having children, particularly at a younger age, offers protection from breast cancer. Each birth is estimated to reduce risk by 7 per cent. Falling birth rates in Western societies account for some of the rise in breast cancer; on average women in the UK now have 1.6 children compared to 2.9 children 40 years ago. Hormonal changes during pregnancy prepare the breast for milk production (even if women do not ultimately breast-feed) and permanently change the structure of the breast. After pregnancy, cells within the milk ducts develop at a much slower rate, which allows more time for any genetic mistakes that may arise to be repaired. Having more children confers greater protection, as each subsequent pregnancy makes breast cells less likely to become damaged.

Pregnancy does not immediately reduce risk. The high circulating levels of hormones (oestrogen and progesterone) during pregnancy can actually stimulate breast cells to grow, and slightly increase risk in the ten years after the first pregnancy especially. This is more of a problem for women who have their first pregnancy later in life, who are more likely to have damaged cells within the breast (and who may have already initiated the development of cancer – see page 33), which are promoted to grow by high levels of hormones during pregnancy. Pregnancy before the age of 30 reduces breast cancer risk; after this age the opposite appears to be true, as each pregnancy after the age of 30 seems to increase breast cancer risk by 3 per cent.

Breast-feeding provides additional breast cancer protection due to the beneficial effects of lactation on the breast and the delay in resumption of normal menstrual cycles. A 2003 overview analysis of 150,000 women published in *The Lancet* showed the longer women breast-feed the more they are protected against breast cancer. Risk decreased by 4.3 per cent for every 12 months of breast-feeding. This adds to the long list of the benefits of breast-feeding

Hormonal and reproductive factors and breast cancer risk

	Effect on risk
Starting periods before age of 11, compared to age of 14	Increased by 30%
No full-term pregnancies	Increased by 30–40%
First full-term pregnancy after the age of 30 years, compared to first pregnancy before age of 30	Increased by 35%
Breast-feeding	Decreased by 4% for each 12 months of breast-feeding
Menopause after the age of 55 years	Increased by 50%
Hormone replacement therapy:	
Current user	Increased by 30–100%
Past user 5–10 years before or more	No effect
Oral contraceptives:	
Current	Increased by 24%
Past user 10 or more years before	No effect

to mother and baby. In the UK only 71 per cent of women attempt breast-feeding at all, many give up within a few weeks and half within four months, which is unlikely to deliver significant cancer protection. The effects of these hormonal reproductive factors on breast cancer risk are summarised in the table above.

Environmental and lifestyle factors

Many women believe that whether they get breast cancer or not is out of their individual control, and that the worldwide epidemic is linked to exposure to many chemicals in the toxic, polluted environment. Certainly a number of chemicals commonly found in food (for example, the pesticide DDT dichlorodiphenyltricholoethane and

PCBs polychlorinated biphenyls), in our homes (parabens in plastics, solvents, deodorants and cleaning fluids) and in the air (polycylic aromatic hydrocarbons – PAH) have been under suspicion of causing breast cancer for some time. Many of these agents pose a legitimate concern as they have oestrogen-like activity (remember that oestrogen stimulates breast cancer), can take many years to break down (DDT metabolite DDE 7–11 years; PCB 5–25 years) and tend to accumulate in fat stores in our bodies, including the breast. Careful studies consistently show that these agents in fact have very weak oestrogen activity, which is considerably less potent than oestrogen naturally in the body (which is itself listed as a known human carcinogen or cancer causing substance in the National Toxicology Programme Report). Most studies have failed to find different levels of toxins in women with and without breast cancer. Doubts remain about the potential combined effects of these chemicals and the effects of exposure to these chemicals in young people.

Despite these unanswered questions the consensus among most scientists who have studied these issues in detail, including researchers at Genesis, is that the toxins that are all too common in the environment are unlikely to impact on the risk of breast cancer. If any risk does exist it is likely to be insignificant compared to the other avoidable risk factors, such as obesity, that are addressed in this book. For the main threat to health, it is suggested that people should instead look within their own bodies. Infinitely higher levels of cancer causing factors are produced within the bodies of people who are overweight and make unwise dietary and lifestyle choices (see page 56). The message is that the risk of breast cancer can be within women's own control. Personal lifestyle choices have a far greater effect on the risk of breast cancer than what is happening in the outside world.

Pesticides and other contaminants in foods
The pesticide DDT, PCBs (used in the production of electrical equipment, paint and paper) and dioxins (by-products of burning fuels) are all found in foods. DDT and PCBs were first used in 1945 and banned in the 1970s but are still present in air, water and soil, and,

along with dioxins, are taken up by feeding animals and fish. These toxins accumulate in fat stores of animals and fish, hence are found in meat, fish and dairy products, particularly the higher fat versions. In 1993 Dr Wolff and colleagues at the Department of Environmental and Occupational Medicine, New York, raised concern by showing two to fourfold higher rates of breast cancer among women with the highest blood levels of DDT and PCB residues.[18] Women can be reassured that with rare exceptions most subsequent studies have not replicated these findings; two studies have even shown higher levels of these toxins to have a protective effect![19] The weak oestrogen effects of these chemicals are nowhere near as much of a threat to health as the oestrogen produced in the body. Furthermore any potential threat from these agents may have been a thing of the past and not relevant today. Since the ban on use intakes of DDT, PCB and dioxins are falling, and are estimated to have reduced by 85 per cent in the past 20 years.

Other pesticides besides DDT are still used on crops or added to crops after harvesting and during storage to preserve foods. Residues of these pesticides are found in foods. These chemicals have all undergone rigorous testing to ensure their safety, so eating these residues is extremely unlikely to cause harm. To put the health risks of pesticide residues into perspective you would have to eat an estimated 12,000 oranges (including their skins) to accumulate a toxic dose of their pesticides. This is hardly a likely scenario, especially as you would have already died from vitamin C toxicity by the time you had eaten 8000 oranges!

Many people instinctively want to limit chemicals in the diet if possible. It is probably prudent to wash or peel fruit and vegetables to help remove dirt and these residues. Some pesticides are actually found within fruit and vegetables, but cooking will remove most of these. You may prefer to choose organic foods, which have lower levels of residues, but are not guaranteed pesticide free (see boxed section on page 48).

Polycyclic hydrocarbons (PCH) are contaminants found in a number of foods such as alcoholic drinks, smoked, cured foods and meat and fish cooked at high temperatures. Most PCH comes from air pollution, such as coal smoke and tobacco smoke, rather than from the diet. Some women may be more susceptible to the effects of these toxins. A recent survey among women living in Long Island in the USA found women who had the highest level of damage to genetic material from exposure to these chemicals were 50 per cent more likely to develop breast cancer than women with minimal damage.[20]

It has been claimed that the chemicals commonly found in food packaging (phthalates), cosmetics and deodorants (parabens) help to cause cancer. Although a recently publicised paper found parabens in breast tumours, there are no population data to support their role in breast cancer,[21] and the dose and weak oestrogen activity of these substances is thought unlikely to pose a cancer risk.[22]

Another concern is the effects of radiation on health. Exposure to high doses of radiation before the age of 30 is known to damage the genetic material in the breast, increasing the likelihood of developing breast cancer. Such exposure is an unlikely occurrence for most women. Two notable exceptions, who do have higher rates of breast cancer, are women who were exposed to high doses of radiation from the atomic bombs dropped on Hiroshima and Nagasaki in Japan at the end of the Second World War, and former Hodgkin's and lymphoma patients who received chest irradiation as children or young women. It has already been stated that the very small dose of radiation from mammograms is not thought to pose a problem (see page 29).

The effects of cosmic radiation from flying on breast cancer risk are not known. Flight attendants do have a slightly higher risk of breast cancer than the rest of the population, but the role of cosmic radiation, disrupted body clock, jet fuel exposure or other lifestyle factors in this is not known.

People worry that exposure to electromagnetic fields from living close to power lines or from electric blankets will increase cancer risk. Electromagnetic fields pose a theoretical risk as they could potentially disrupt the menstrual cycle by reducing melatonin production from the pituitary gland, and increasing levels of the cancer promoting hormones prolactin and oestrogen. However, there is no good evidence to link these exposures to breast cancer risk.

Organic versus conventional and GM crops

Many people choose to eat organic foods as a way of reducing pesticides in the diet and because they believe organic foods to be more nutritious than conventionally grown produce. Existing evidence however suggests that a well-balanced diet can equally improve health, regardless of its organic, conventional or indeed genetically modified (GM) origin.

Organic food is produced by growers who are registered and approved by organic certification bodies (such as the Soil Association in the UK). Land has to have been farmed organically for the conversion period (normally two years) before food can be sold as 'organic' and organic food cannot contain harmful hydrogenated (or hardened) fats (see page 83). Organic foods are not free of chemicals and pesticides but are grown with the use of a limited range of approved products. Typically organic food has one-sixth of the pesticide residue dose found in conventionally grown foods. Organic food may still be contaminated with organic chlorine pesticides such as DDT, which persist in the environment, and small amounts occur in 10 per cent of organic foods.[23]

Many people assume organic food to be more nutritious, which is the case for some but by no means all organic food. A recent report from the Soil Association summarised evidence comparing the vitamin and mineral (calcium, magnesium, iron and chromium) content of organic and conventionally grown fruits and vegetables; seven studies found the organic versions to be superior, six studies found no difference between the foods and one found conventional food to be superior.[24]

Genetically modified (GM) food has had lots of publicity since its first commercial production in the UK in 1996. GM technology involves identifying one or several genes, which provide a desired characteristic, that are introduced into the genetic material of a crop plant. Foods that come from a GM crop are termed 'GM ingredients' if the genetic material (DNA) is present in the food, or 'GM derived ingredients' if the DNA is removed from the final food as it is with soya oil, or 'GM processing aid' when a GM organism (such as bacteria) is used to make a product without GM material being present in the ingredients or the final product.

Some of the specific fears expressed by opponents of GM technology include alteration in nutritional quality of foods, potential toxicity and possible antibiotic resistance from GM crops, potential allergenicity and carcinogenicity from consuming GM foods. In addition, some more general concerns include environmental pollution, unintentional gene transfer to wild plants, possible creation of new viruses and toxins, and threat to crop genetic diversity. GM food is routinely assessed for safety and there is currently no evidence that consuming DNA from GM foods will have an adverse effect on health.

The environmental and ethical issues (plus or minus) surrounding organic, GM and conventional foods are beyond the scope of this book.

Smoking

Most people are well aware of the strong links between smoking and cancer, particularly with lung cancer. You are probably wondering why smoking has not yet been mentioned in the context of breast cancer. Cigarettes contain more than 50 identifiable cancer causing substances and account for about one-fifth of cancers worldwide, particularly cancers of the mouth, throat, oesophagus (gullet), pancreas, cervix, bladder and leukaemia. However, smoking only has weak links with breast cancer, although there is some evidence that women who start smoking at a younger age and who smoke heavily for many years may increase their risk by 30 per cent.[25] Smoking during pregnancy and passive smoking may also increase risk.[19] Even among these women the effects of smoking on breast cancer are by no means as great as the increase in risk linked to weight gain, which can be as much as double.

An estimated one in five women may be particularly susceptible to the effects of smoking as they have genes that convert the toxic chemicals in tobacco to their active cancer causing forms; if these women smoke they are three to 13 times as likely to develop breast cancer.[26]

Clearly, smoking is bad for your health – half the people who smoke will die prematurely as a result of it! If you currently smoke the best thing for the sake of your health and the health of your family is to stop. Giving up smoking can be a difficult challenge. There is no substitute for will-power but lots of resources and services are now available to help people quit. Advice from a trained professional such as a nurse, GP or smoking counsellor can help you stop smoking. Your GP may be able to prescribe aids such as nicotine patches and medication such as bupropion, and may recommend services in your area that provide one-to-one counselling. There are also many Stop Smoking groups (see the Resources section).

Stress

Many people have stressful, hectic lifestyles. Stress is certainly not good for physical and mental health, but contrary to what many may think there is little to suggest that stress puts women at higher risk of breast cancer. If anything, some evidence points to chronic low key stress making women less likely to get the disease. A 2005 study published in the *British Medical Journal* assessed levels of stress in nearly 7000 Danish women in the Copenhagen City Heart Study, and followed them for 18 years. Surprisingly, women with the highest reported levels of stress were 40 per cent less likely to get breast cancer. These findings most likely reflected lower levels of oestrogen in the women who were chronically stressed.[27] The authors of the study were quick to point out that stress was over-all bad for health, and that more of the most stressed women actually died from other causes. Stress is linked to conditions such as heart disease, depression and even osteoporosis. What's more, high levels of the stress hormone cortisol do not cause weight gain, but encourage any fat put on to be laid down around the abdomen, which is potentially the most harmful fat for health.

Chronic stress is also well known to suppress the immune system, which offers a defence against infections and many diseases. This may increase susceptibility to certain cancers such as blood cancers, lymphoma, skin cancer, bladder cancer and cancer of the cervix. Stress is not thought to be a risk factor for breast cancer in that there is no good evidence that the immune system seeks out and defends the body from growing tumour cells in the breast, unlike the cancers mentioned above. Women who have been diagnosed with breast cancer need not fear that stressful life experiences will precipitate the return of their disease. Stress does not appear to increase chances of relapse from breast cancer,[28] although stress reducing strategies are recommended for the general well-being of all women who have been diagnosed with breast cancer.

Clearly it is important to manage stress and not let it rule your life. Before you can do this you need to identify the stressors in your life, learn to recognise the symptoms and acknowledge the stress in your life. The list of possible stressors is endless but may include:
• work-related issues
• family issues, such as children, partners, acting as a carer for older or sick relatives
• bereavement, loss, separation

- juggling many roles
- not enough time
- feeling you are spread too thinly
- pace of life
- fear of failure
- lack of support
- feelings of guilt if you take time out
- diet, weight, exercise and health issues.

Next, be aware of the signs of stress. Common signs include feeling that you can't switch off, not coping as well as usual, not being as efficient, feeling wound up, panicked, unable to support others, feeling you are letting people down, feeling tired, having problems sleeping and having a short fuse. You may find yourself eating more or sometimes less, or drinking more alcohol.

Acknowledging stress is the most important step you can take in coping with it. The best coping strategy for you is of course a personal issue. Many people turn to food and drink when they are stressed, and this is of course a major factor in weight problems. It is far better to manage stress with strategies that are not food related. You may find having a massage or aromatherapy treatment helpful; even a simple hand massage can have deeply relaxing effects. Another bonus for the dieter is that these treatments act as an appetite suppressant due to toxins that are released during the treatment. Take time to think how you might help yourself. The list below was suggested by women from one of the Genesis research studies and may offer some good ideas:

- pampering yourself with a massage or a facial
- looking for support by talking, socialising with friends or family
- writing lists, keeping a diary, recreating order
- having time out, holidays
- making time to exercise, being outdoors, especially in the sunshine, gardening
- escapism, such as reading a good book, watching television, a good film, jigsaws, listening to relaxing music
- having a good cry, scream or laugh
- having a rest, lie down, relaxation tapes, yoga

- having sex
- being near or in water, swimming, baths, showers, sauna, steam room, flotation tank
- burning aromatherapy oils known for their relaxing properties, such as bergamot, camomile, clary sage, frankincense, lavender, neroli rose, ylang ylang
- making time for hobbies, pets, wildlife watching.

Summary

- *Only 5 per cent of breast cancers are due to readily identifiable inherited genes. This means that 90 to 95 per cent of breast cancers are the result of hormones, lifestyle and the environment.*

- *Risk of breast cancer goes up as women get older.*

- *Breast cancer can begin to develop many years before it is detected. Sensible lifestyle choices throughout life can reduce the risk of breast cancer.*

- *The breast cancer susceptibility genes BRCA1 and BRCA2 are rare, only occurring in two out of every 1000 women in Western countries.*

- *Inheriting the BRCA1 or BRCA2 gene does not mean that cancer is inevitable; about 30 per cent of gene carriers will not develop breast cancer.*

- *Women with BRCA genes and family history of the disease should make sensible lifestyle choices to reduce their risk of cancer, as well as considering risk reduction surgery.*

- *Environmental factors such as pesticides and chemicals are not likely to be a major cause of breast cancer. High levels of cancer causing factors and hormones produced within the bodies of people who are overweight and make unwise dietary and lifestyle choices pose a far greater threat to their health.*

- *Smoking and stress are bad for the general health but do not have strong links with breast cancer.*

'What's my current risk of breast cancer?'

GAUGING YOUR CURRENT CANCER RISK is a critical step towards helping you decide how and by how much you will be likely to reduce it. You have already seen how a number of factors affect breast cancer risk, including age, age at first period, number of children, weight gain and family history. Breast cancer may occur in families due to chance, shared environmental/lifestyle risk factors or to increased genetic susceptibility. A woman's risk increases according to the number of first degree relatives (mothers or sisters) who have developed breast cancer. The probability of a woman aged 20 developing breast cancer by the age of 80 who has no relatives affected with breast cancer is 8 per cent (one chance in 13); one affected relative, 13 per cent (one in eight); and two affected relatives, 20 per cent (one in five). Also, the risk of developing breast cancer is greater in women the younger their relative was when she developed the disease. A woman with one relative diagnosed under the age of 40 has a risk of 20 per cent (one in five), which is the same risk as a woman who has two affected first degree relatives of a later age.

Having read this far, you will already be aware that weight gain dramatically increases risk. Women who have gained 3 stone (19 kilograms) in weight since the age of 20 have a lifetime risk of one in five. As you can see from the table on page 57, having this extra weight is worse than having no children and worse than taking HRT for ten years. It is equivalent to having a mother or sister with breast cancer aged younger than 40 years or having two relatives diagnosed at older ages. It is worse than having one close relative diagnosed aged over 40 years of age. You cannot do anything about your family history but you can do something about your weight. It was described earlier (see page 33) how the beginnings of cancer may have already started to develop within the breast, so losing weight in your 30s, 40s, 50s or even 60s is a good time to stop the cancer from developing any further. Just think, if you can lose this excess weight you can reduce your risk, maybe back down to one in ten, the normal risk in the population. In other words you can nearly halve what would have been your projected risk.

The table opposite shows how breast cancer risk is affected by various factors. However, predicting who will actually get breast cancer with any degree of certainty is extremely difficult even when the many factors that need to be taken into account are included. Doctors working in prevention clinics use a number of prediction programmes to estimate risk based on known family history and lifestyle factors. The best programme is the Tyrer Cuzick model developed by Professor Jack Cuzick and Jonathon Tyrer from Cancer Research UK Department of Epidemiology, Mathematics and Statistics. This programme is able to predict who is likely to get breast cancer with 75 per cent accuracy. This means three-quarters of the women who develop breast cancer will be correctly identified, but also means that the remaining 25 per cent would not.

A few web-based assessment tools are also available. The best of these is found on the Harvard Center for Cancer Prevention website (see Resources on page 276), which asks you to enter details of your family history, current weight, height, diet, use of hormones, number of children and medical history, though not body fat or weight gain. The programme will tell you whether you are average, high or low risk. Don't forget that these programmes can only provide a rough estimate of risk; being a low risk does not guarantee you'll never get cancer.

Factors influencing risk of breast cancer*

Factor	Population	Risk
Taking OC for 10 years from 30–40 years	1 chance in 10	10%
Taking combined HRT from 50–60 years	1 chance in 7	14%
Having no children	1 chance in 6	16%
Gaining 1 stone (6.3 kg) since the age of 20	1 chance in 8	13%
Gaining 2 stone (12.7 kg) since the age of 20	1 chance in 6	16%
Gaining 3 stone (19 kg) since the age of 20	1 chance in 5	20%
Having a mother or sister who were diagnosed aged over 40 years of age	1 chance in 8	13%
Having a mother or sister who were diagnosed at less than 40 years of age	1 chance in 5	20%
Having 2 close relatives who were diagnosed aged over 40 years of age	1 chance in 5	20%

Key: OC = oral contraceptives; HRT = hormone replacement therapy
* figues for the UK

Lifestyle and breast cancer risk – putting you in control

A number of factors that increase the risk of breast cancer, such as a fault in genes, age and to a certain extent if and when you have children, are out of your control. The good news is that there are lifestyle choices well within your control, which have a profound effect on your risk of breast cancer. What you eat, how much you exercise and above all what you weigh are lifestyle choices that have a great impact on your personal risk of breast cancer. It is estimated that a quarter of breast cancer cases worldwide could be

Anne-Marie's story

Anne-Marie is a 39-year-old single working mum, with a 5-year-old son. There is a history of ovarian and breast cancer in Anne-Marie's family: her mother and aunt succumbed respectively to ovarian and breast cancer at only 53 years of age, when Anne-Marie was in her mid 20s. She is estimated to have a one in three chance of developing breast cancer. Anne-Marie has been coming to the family history clinic for 6 years for regular cancer screening and is determined to do all she can to stay well and make sure that her son does not have to the endure the anguish of seeing her suffer with cancer. Until Anne-Marie was recruited to our weight loss research study, she confesses to not thinking much about lifestyle in relation to her cancer risk. In common with her mother, Anne-Marie had struggled with her weight throughout her adult life, weighing 14 stone (89 kg) when she married in her late 20s. This increased to 15½ stone (96 kg) following her pregnancy and comfort eating due to the strain of divorce. After 12 months of following the diet and exercise plan Anne-Marie had lost a massive 26 pounds (12 kg) of body fat, 6½ inches (17 cm) from her waist, 8 inches (20 cm) from her hips and 8 inches (20 cm) from her bust. The previously raised levels of insulin and fats in her blood had halved, and this, along with other hormonal changes (a 22 per cent drop in testosterone), are likely to further reduce her cancer risk.

'The diet plans are easy to follow, and are based on sensible everyday foods, which means I can make sure my boy eats healthily, too. Keeping a food diary made me realise just what, and importantly how much, I normally ate. My diet was quite healthy, but my portion sizes had grown out of control. Previous slimming attempts have been short lived but I have managed to keep the weight off with a healthy diet plan for nearly 3 years now. I rarely miss my 3-weekly hour-long training sessions at the gym – it's part of my social life. Knowing the health reasons for weight loss has been a great motivator for me. Of course I have the occasional treat food, sometimes at the weekend, but make sure I get quickly back on track.'

prevented if people controlled their weight and were more active. Certainly weight control and exercise have at least as much or a greater effect on risk than do the hormonal risk factors. The recent concerns over the links between HRT and breast cancer have received a lot of publicity. Interestingly HRT does not pose a threat to health soon after stopping treatment. Likewise, excess weight and lack of exercise have a detrimental effect on our health as long as they prevail. Successful weight reduction or taking up regular exercise will immediately work at reducing this excess risk.

Summary

- *A woman's risk increases according to the number of first degree relatives who have developed breast cancer.*

- *What you eat, how much you exercise and above all what you weigh have a great impact on your personal risk of breast cancer.*

- *The Pill and HRT increase the risk of breast cancer while they are taken and up to ten years after stopping.*

- *Having children before the age of 30 and breast-feeding both lower breast cancer risk.*

PART TWO

The Importance of a Healthy Lifestyle

Excess weight and increased breast cancer risk

EVERYONE KNOWS that eating too many calories, lack of exercise, or most usually both, lead to weight gain. You may not have been aware before reading this book that eating too many calories, lack of exercise and putting on weight also increase a woman's risk of developing breast cancer. It was stated earlier that breast cancer can start to develop many years before it is detected (see page 25). There is good evidence that eating too many calories, being sedentary and putting on weight throughout our lives, in other words during childhood, adolescence and during both the pre and post-menopausal years can each increase a woman's chances of developing breast cancer.

Weight in the early years

It is obviously difficult to link what is eaten by a child to the detection of a cancer in that child many years later. Despite this, several lines of evidence suggest that weight and diet and exercise habits in these early years may impact on the risk of developing breast cancer later in life. It has already been mentioned that starting periods at an early age increases the risk of breast cancer. Over the past century there has been a trend for girls in Western societies to begin their periods earlier. Back in the 1840s girls started their periods on average between the ages of 16 and 17. Today in the West, periods start on average at the age of 12 or 13. Girls in rural China still typically start periods at the age of 17. This earlier onset of periods is thought to be linked to higher weights, larger stores of body fat and low levels of exercise among Western girls today compared to their predecessors. These factors all increase blood levels of the hormone leptin to rise above a critical level, which triggers the reproductive system to become active. Research from the Ohio State University in the USA tracked 343 girls and found each additional kilogram (2.2 pounds) of fat in girls lowered the age that they started their periods by one year.[1]

Breast tissue may be particularly vulnerable to cancer causing agents such as high levels of hormones and toxins during adolescence, as the breast tissue is undergoing rapid growth at this time. Growth spurts during adolescence, linked to higher levels of growth factors, increase risk and probably account for observations that women who are taller than 5 foot 9 inches (1.75 metres) have a 25 to 40 per cent greater breast cancer risk than women who are shorter than 5 foot 3 inches (1.6 metres).[2]

Women who experienced puberty during times of food rationing and calorie restriction in Norway during the Second World War subsequently had 13 per cent less breast cancer in later life than women with normal food supplies, suggesting that calorie intake during puberty affects later risk of breast cancer.[3] Though it may be difficult to convince 'immortal' children and teenagers that what they eat and weigh will affect their risk of disease later in life, they should be nevertheless encouraged to adopt healthy eating and exercise behaviours.

Weight gain during adult life

Gains in weight and inches on the waistline are considered an inevitable part of getting older within Western societies. On average, women in the UK, Australia and New Zealand gain 1 stone (6.3 kilograms) in weight and about 6 inches (15 centimetres) on their waistline over adult life. This weight gain is not an inevitable part of ageing, but instead an inevitable result of people becoming more sedentary as they get older, but failing to moderate dietary intake accordingly. National data highlight the fact that women actually gain the majority of weight between the ages of 20 and 50, in other

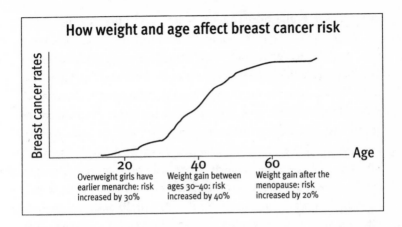

How weight and age affect breast cancer risk

Breast cancer rates

Age

20
Overweight girls have
earlier menarche: risk
increased by 30%

40
Weight gain between
ages 30–40: risk
increased by 40%

60
Weight gain after the
menopause: risk
increased by 20%

words long before they reach the menopause. Weight problems clearly do not, as many people believe, only start after the menopause – they have already happened!

What many women probably also don't realise is the large health risk, and the dramatic increase in breast cancer risk, which accompanies these gains in weight and girth. Experts agree that weight gain throughout adult life is a major risk factor for breast cancer. Twelve good quality studies have consistently highlighted strong links between weight gain and breast cancer risk. One study that highlights the perils of weight gain after the age of 18 comes from Dr Huang from the Harvard School of Public Health in Boston in the USA. This study followed 95,256 nurses for 16 years to see which factors were linked to the development of breast cancer. Women who had gained just 1 stone (6.3 kilograms) in weight since the age of 18 were 30 per cent more likely to develop breast cancer, which occurred in one out of eight of these women. Women who had gained more than 3 stone (19 kilograms) in weight since the age of 18 doubled their risk of breast cancer, which occurred in one in five of these women![4]

Putting on weight is clearly bad news for breast cancer risk. An interesting question is whether weight gain at different stages of life has different effects on risk, in other words, does putting on weight between the ages of 18 and 30 have different effects compared to putting on weight between the ages of 30 and 50 or after the menopause? Is the breast more or less susceptible to the cancer causing effects of weight gain at different times of life? To answer this question we undertook a collaborative study with Professor Tom Sellers and his team of scientists at the University of Minnesota in the USA, using data collected from 33,000 healthy women living in Iowa, in the Iowa Women's Health Study. Women in the study had carefully documented how their weight had changed throughout adult life and were followed up for 16 years, during which time nearly 2000 of the women developed breast cancer. The study clearly showed weight gain was bad news for breast cancer risk, particularly if it was gained between the ages of 30 and 50. The lowest rates were seen in women whose weight had not changed (254 women). Gaining at least ½ stone (3.2 kilograms) between the ages of 18 to 30 only increased risk by 5 per cent (only estimated to cause eight extra cases of breast cancer), gaining at least ½ stone (3.2 kilograms) after the menopause increased risk by 20 per cent (led to 42 extra cases), while weight gain from 30 to 50 increased risk by 30 per cent (and was responsible for an estimated 72 extra cases of breast cancer). The clear message from these studies is that women of any age should watch their weight. Women aged 30 to 50 should be especially vigilant as this is a time when they are very likely to put on weight and when the breast appears most susceptible to the cancer promoting effects of weight gain and high calorie intakes.[5] Damage that may have already occurred within breast tissue by the age of 30 could be promoted to develop into a cancer in the presence of high energy intakes and higher circulating hormone levels over these years before the menopause.

Although gaining weight after the menopause is less common it also increases risk of breast cancer. After the menopause the body's main source of oestrogen is from body fat stores. It has already been explained that oestrogen is one of the main hormones that encourages breast cancer to develop and grow. Weight gain after the menopause appears to promote cancer because of its oestrogen effects. Weight gain does not seem to be as much of a risk factor for women who are currently or who have recently taken hormone replacement therapy (HRT). HRT will of course increase levels of oestrogen in the body regardless of a women's weight, thus HRT removes the normal variation in oestrogen levels due to body weight.

Why does weight gain cause breast cancer?
Gains in body fat

Body weight is determined by the amount of bone, muscle, water and fat in the body. Since weight gain reflects gains in body fat for most people, the increase in breast cancer risk with weight gain is actually due to gains in body fat. Many people think fat is just harmless padding. Scientists also held this view until the mid 1990s when a number of ground-breaking discoveries revealed the pivotal role of fat in producing a number of key hormones. It is now known that fat is an active tissue containing fat cells, which produce over 20 hormones and other factors that regulate many systems in the body, including the menstrual cycle, bones and blood pressure. Thin people have some fat cells, which are small and which produce the correct balance of these hormones and factors to promote good health. Fatter people may have a few more fat cells, but the key difference is that heavier people have larger, fat-filled fat cells, which behave differently to the smaller cells found in thinner people. These enlarged fat cells lose their ability to regulate production of hormones and produce greater amounts of hormones and also growth factors, which are at high enough levels to promote cancer. Inflammatory cells, known as macrophages, are also recruited into these large fat cells, which subsequently release inflammatory factors in the bloodstream leading to a low grade level of inflammation throughout the body. This inflammation in turn prevents insulin working efficiently, leading to insulin resistance and higher circulating levels of cancer promoting insulin. Both low grade inflammation and insulin resistance can promote the development of cancer (see page 69) and are linked to heart disease (see page 99).

You will recall that fat is the main production site of oestrogen (the major cancer promoting hormone) after the menopause (see page 37). Fat cells are also the major site for production of the hormone leptin, which is well known to promote the growth and spread of breast cancer. Fat cells are also responsible for production of the recently discovered hormone adiponectin, which importantly halts the spread of cancer. This is actually produced in reduced amounts by larger fat cells in fatter people and increases when weight is lost, which is why cancers can be more likely to spread in heavier people.

From reading all the above, you should start to be convinced that large fat stores can promote cancers to develop, grow and spread, and you probably already know that they are linked to many other common diseases such as heart disease, diabetes and stroke.

The reading on the scales is not always the best way to tell if you are a healthy weight. People who do a lot of exercise may appear to be heavier because they have a higher muscle mass. A healthy weight is when the body has the right amount of fat stores, and for women the figure is between 20 and 28 per cent of their body weight as fat. High levels of body fat increase breast cancer risk. A closer look at the amounts of fat in 12,000 women in the Malmö Diet and Cancer Study in Sweden revealed that breast cancer was twice as likely in women who had 36 per cent or more of their body as fat, compared to women with less than 27 per cent of their body as fat.[6]

Having too little body fat is also bad for your health. Less than 20 per cent of weight as fat can disrupt normal menstrual cycles in premenopausal women and can lead to very low oestrogen levels in post-menopausal women. Admittedly, lower levels of oestrogen may be helpful from a breast cancer standpoint, but could predispose these lighter women to thin bones and osteoporosis, and may even increase the likelihood of dementia later in life.

Amounts of body fat can be assessed from special medical scans (DEXA scans) or, more commonly, using bioelectrical impedance meters. These send a small, safe electrical signal through the body, which can discern the difference between fat and muscle and provide an accurate reading based on impedance, weight, age, height and gender. Bathroom scales or hand-held versions of impedance meters are commercially available.

A simple way to assess your body fat is to use the Genesis Body Fat Ready Reckoner on pages 72–73, which estimates your body fat from your weight, height and hip measurements. This scale was based on research findings from our research on premenopausal women, for whom it probably works best. The increasing tendency for older women to carry fat around their abdomens, may mean the scale could slightly underestimate levels of body fat in older women.

You may have heard about healthy weight in terms of healthy body mass index (BMI). Body mass index is calculated as your weight (in kilograms) divided by height (in metres) squared. For example, the average woman in the UK weighs 70 kilograms (11 stone) and is 1.61 metres (5 foot 3½ inches) tall, which means she has a BMI of 27.

$$BMI = \frac{weight}{(height \times height)} \qquad BMI = \frac{70}{(1.61 \times 1.61)} = 27$$

If you don't want to do the maths, you will find a BMI table on page 266. The normal range of BMI is 18.5 to 25. The average woman in the UK falls in the range 25 to 29. This is overweight and a threat to health. BMI of 30 or greater is defined as obese and a major threat to health. The healthiest level BMI is actually around 20. Risk of cancer and many other diseases gradually increases above this, and the higher you go the higher your risk. However, while BMI is a useful benchmark for assessing your weight, it is not a great predictor of breast cancer risk. It is much better to assess whether or not you have a healthy fat level.

Watch your waistline

Most people have some fat around their middles that they can pinch, the so-called subcutaneous fat, but you may not be aware that fat is also stored within the abdomen, around the organs. This 'intra abdominal fat' is an important source of the cancer promoting hormones oestrogen and testosterone. Enlarged fat cells within the abdomen are the most likely of any of the fat cells stored in the body to recruit inflammatory cells and release inflammatory factors causing low grade inflammation throughout the body (see page 67). The hormone insulin, which helps to control the levels of sugar in the blood, has been shown to play a part in the growth of breast cancer when present at higher levels in the body. Fat reserves in the abdomen interfere with the body's ability to use insulin, which subsequently builds up to higher levels. These higher insulin levels may also directly promote cancer growth or may increase cancer risk by boosting the activity of oestrogen and testosterone. Both these hormones are either carried around the blood-stream by carrier proteins (sex hormone binding proteins) or can circulate freely in the body in more active cancer promoting forms. More insulin means fewer carrier proteins are produced, which increases the potential cancer promoting power of these hormones. A waist measurement of 32 inches (80 centimetres) or more puts women (non-Asian, see below) at moderate risk of having high insulin levels, while a waist measurement of 35 inches (88 centimetres) or more places at women at a substantially increased risk. For women of South Asian descent a waist of 32 inches (80 centimetres) or more is associated with a substantially increased risk.

It is a worrying fact that 30 to 40 per cent of adults in developed countries have raised levels of insulin. Aside from causing extra fat around the abdomen, a diet high in saturated fat and refined carbohydrates can elevate insulin levels. Regular exercise, wholegrain foods and an adequate supply of chromium all help control insulin

Waist measurement	Conclusion	Recommendations
32 in (80 cm) or less all women	Healthy waist	Avoid any future increases in your waist
32–35 in (80–88 cm) non-Asian	At increased health risk	Try to reduce your waist
32–35 in (80–88 cm) Asian	High risk to health	Need to reduce your waist
35 in (88 cm) or more all women	High risk to health	Need to reduce your waist

levels. Good food sources of chromium include lean meat, whole grains (such as wholemeal bread and whole oats), lentils and spices.

Most women tend to gain weight around the hips and thighs during adolescence and in their 20s. There are variations between people, but by and large fat accumulates around the abdomen during pregnancy and in women after the age of 30. Waist measurement is a good proxy of the amount of fat stored around the abdomen. Given the adverse effect abdominal fat has on the balance of hormones in the body, as outlined above, it will not surprise you to learn that having a large waist can increase your risk of breast cancer. Our 2003 overview paper published in *Obesity Review*, based on 105,000 women and nearly 4000 cases of breast cancer, showed having a bigger waist put women at higher risk of breast cancer. After the menopause bigger waist measurements seem to increase risk as women with bigger waists generally carried more weight over their bodies. Interestingly for younger women, weight specifically carried around the waist seemed to be particularly linked to risk. Whatever their age, women with a waist measurement of 36 inches (90 centimetres) or more had a 40 per cent greater risk of breast cancer compared to women with waist of 29 inches (73 centimetres).[7]

Too many calories can cause cancer

Most people know that eating too many calories puts on weight but most people probably don't realise that just consuming too many calories (regardless of the foods they come from) is in itself enough to promote cancer to develop, grow and spread.

It has already been explained how highly unstable molecules known as free radicals are produced as a by-product of digestion and processing any food that we eat. Eating too much of any food and too many calories is therefore one of the major causes of the production of free radicals in the body. If you recall from page 26, damage to genetic material from these unstable molecules within the breast cells can be the first step in the development of breast cancer, so eating too much can easily kick-start the cancer process.

High calorie intakes can promote cancers to grow and spread by escalating levels of hormones such as oestrogen, progesterone,

(continued on page 74)

Do you have a healthy body fat level?

GENESIS BODY FAT READY RECKONER

Follow these five simple steps to estimate your percentage body fat:

1. Weigh yourself on reliable scales.
2. Estimate your body mass index (BMI) using the formula on page 69 or use the BMI chart on page 266.
3. While standing and breathing out, measure your hips, in inches, at the widest point over your buttocks (to convert centimetres to inches, divide by 2.54).
4. Look up your BMI and hip measurements in the columns opposite to find the corresponding constants A and B.
5. Add constants A and B then subtract 11. This will give you an estimate of your percentage body fat.

For example, if you have a BMI of 28 and a hip measurement of 44 inches (112 centimetres), then your percentage body fat will be 37.

A BMI of 28 gives a Constant A of 25; 44 inch hips give a Constant B of 23

Percentage body fat = 25 + 23 − 11

Percentage body fat = 37

The actual amount of fat in pounds can be estimated from your percentage fat and weight

Actual fat = % fat ÷ 100 x weight in lb

For example, if your percentage body fat is 37 and you weigh 12 stone i.e. 168 lb then the amount of actual fat is 62 lb

Actual fat (lb) = (37/100) x 168

Actual fat (lb) = 62 lb (28 kg)

Body Mass Index	Constant A	Hips – inches	Constant B
18	16	30	16
19	17	31	16
20	18	32	17
21	18	33	17
22	19	34	18
23	20	35	18
24	21	36	19
25	22	37	19
26	23	38	20
27	24	39	20
28	25	40	21
29	25	41	21
30	26	42	22
31	27	43	22
32	28	44	23
33	29	45	23
34	30	46	24
35	31	47	24
36	32	48	25
37	32	49	25
38	33	50	26
39	34	51	27
40	35	52	27
41	36	53	28
42	37	54	28
43	38	55	29
44	39	56	29
45	39	57	30
46	40	58	30
47	41	59	31
48	42	60	31

growth factors and inflammatory factors in the blood-stream, and the production of cancer causing factors by fat cells within the breast. High energy (calorie) intakes also act directly on the control centre in the cells to make them more likely to become unrestrained and more likely to multiply, spread and become cancerous. Given the alarming array of cancer promoting effects of high calorie intake, it is little wonder that a 2005 survey among 50,000 Canadian women found those routinely eating more than 2400 calories per day were 45 per cent more likely to develop breast cancer than women who ate fewer than 1600 calories per day.[8]

Weight control, weight loss and breast cancer

Given that weight gain has such a dramatic effect on risk, it follows that avoiding weight gain is the best way to limit your risk of breast cancer. For example, women whose weight remains the same between the age of 18 and 50 are half as likely to develop cancer compared to women who gained 3 stone (19 kilograms). Women who actually lost weight between the age of 18 and 50 in the Iowa Women's Health Study of 33,000 women (not a common occurrence) had the lowest rates, and only one-third of the cancers compared to women who gained weight. Women who lose weight as they get older are quite unusual, so the small numbers who actually lost weight in the study make it difficult to draw firm conclusions.

For women who have already gained weight, all is not lost. Thankfully, the Iowa analysis showed that losing just a few pounds can dramatically reduce your risk. The study also showed the benefits of losing weight at any point in your life. If you are currently younger than 50 years of age, losing just ½ stone (3.2 kilograms) and keeping this off means your risk of breast cancer is 40 per cent lower than it would be if you continued to put on weight. If you have already gone through the menopause, losing at least ½ stone (3.2 kilograms) in weight after the menopause and keeping this off means your risk of breast cancer is some 20 per cent lower than it would be if you continued to put weight on.

How might weight loss reduce risk?

As already mentioned, heavier women have higher circulating levels of cancer promoting hormones such as oestrogen, progesterone, testosterone and insulin. These higher levels of unbound or free hormones are more likely to be taken up by breast cells where they can stimulate cancer growth (see page 37). The large fat cells in heavier women also release greater amounts of cancer promoters into the blood-stream, such as the hormone leptin, together with inflammatory factors (see page 69).

Weight loss helps to correct these imbalances. A recent weight loss study showed weight loss of less than 5 per cent of body weight (at least ½ stone/3.2 kilograms) caused blood levels of testosterone and insulin to fall by 25 per cent and levels of cancer protective sex hormone binding globulin to rise by 25 per cent.[9] Inflammatory markers in the blood fell by 7 per cent. This potentially lowers the exposure of the breast cells to cancer promoting hormones.

Summary

- *25 per cent of all breast cancer cases worldwide are due to excess weight, obesity and a sedentary lifestyle.*

- *Gaining more than 3 stone (19 kilograms) in weight since the age of 20 doubles your risk of developing breast cancer after the menopause.*

- *Women whose weight remains steady, or who lose at least ½ stone (3.2 kilograms) in weight between the ages of 30 and 50, have 40 per cent less breast cancer risk than women who gain weight over this period.*

- *Women whose bodies comprise 36 per cent fat or greater have double the risk of women who have less than 27 per cent of their weight as fat.*

- *Women whose waist measures 36 inches (90 cm) or greater have 40 per cent higher risk of breast cancer than women with waists measuring 29 inches (73 cm) or less.*

The vital ingredients of a healthy diet

THE SEARCH FOR FOODS THAT WILL PROTECT US from cancer is like the search for the Holy Grail. This quest has been avidly pursued over the past 40 years since the pivotal publication by Richard Doll, which suggested that 30 per cent of cancers were related to diet. As you have probably gathered by now cancer is a complex process that develops over many years and goes through many stages. It is highly unlikely that breast cancer will either be caused or prevented by one single food or nutrient.

A number of foods and nutrients appear to have small effects on increased risk but the main culprits seem to be eating too many calories, lack of exercise and, above all, putting on weight. Protection from cancer relates to an overall effect of what you eat.

Alcohol intake and breast cancer risk

Most people know that drinking too much is bad for the health, but most people have also heard that small amounts of alcohol are good for the health. Just what are the benefits and risks of alcohol?

Alcohol misuse is linked to about 22,000 deaths each year in England alone. Modest drinking (one or two drinks a day) is often recommended to protect against heart disease. This recommendation has not been rigorously examined in trials in the same way as, for example, drugs are tested. Doctors do not recommend beginning or increasing drinking habits to improve the health. Some scientists remain sceptical that alcohol is truly heart protective; a 2005 study from the National

Center for Chronic Disease Prevention in Atlanta in the USA suggested that healthier modest drinkers in earlier studies may have had less heart disease for other reasons, apart from their drinking habits.[10] One thing that *is* known is that even modest drinking can increase your risk of breast cancer. The clear message from the 2002 report, Alcohol, Tobacco and Breast Cancer (published in the *British Journal of Cancer*, November 2002) was that each additional unit of alcohol (see section opposite) consumed on a daily basis increases the risk of breast cancer by 7 per cent. If you think you have a particularly high breast cancer risk (see page 57 on estimating your risk), you should probably think about limiting your alcohol intake. Alcohol is thought to promote breast cancer by making breast tissue more susceptible to damage, and by increasing levels of cancer causing hormones oestrogen and testosterone in the blood, particularly in women who are taking hormone replacement therapy. Drinkers also tend to have lower levels of folic acid through low intakes, poorer absorption or altered processing. Data from three large population studies, the US Nurses' Health Study, the Canadian National Breast Screening Study and the Melbourne Collaborative Cohort Study in Australia, suggest that women drinking more than one to two drinks a day were at higher risk of breast cancer, but seemed to be protected if they also consumed a daily 400–600 µg/day folic acid supplement.[11-13] Thus it seems that folic acid may offset some of the harmful effects of alcohol. So, if you drink alcohol you should try to consume plenty of foods rich in folic acid, such as green leafy vegetables, beans, pulses, nuts, seeds, wholegrain cereals and offal, such as kidney and liver. A daily supplement providing 400 µg/day of folic acid may also be advisable. Don't forget that alcohol is fattening as well.

Other drinks

Many people love a cup of tea or coffee and wrongly assume it would be healthier to have decaffeinated versions or not to include these at all. Recent research indicates tea and coffee, caffeinated or otherwise, is not a health hazard; on the contrary, they are packed with antioxidant polyphenols, which can potentially cut the risk of cancer and heart disease.

What's in a drink?

Health recommendations for alcohol often quote safe limits in terms of units. Units are not drinks; in the UK a unit is the amount of alcoholic drink that contains 10 grams of alcohol. When units were first introduced wine was about 8.5 per cent alcohol, so the standard 125-ml drink contained about 10 grams of alcohol, i.e. approximately 1 unit. Most drinks now contain several units of alcohol. For example, a large 250-ml (just under ½ pint) glass of red wine now gives you three-and-a-half units!

Use the table below to work out your daily alcohol intake. Bear in mind that each additional unit you regularly drink can push your cancer risk up by 7 per cent.

Drink	Amount	Size (ml)	% alcohol by volume (Abv)	Units
Red wine	large glass	250	14	3.5
	medium glass	175	14	2.5
	small glass	125	14	1.8
White wine	large glass	250	12	2.7
	medium glass	175	12	2.1
	small glass	125	12	1.5
Champagne	flute	100	12	1.2
Alcopop	bottle	275	5	1.5
Beer	½ pint	284	4.7	1.3
Lager	bottle	330	5	1.6
Cider	½ pint	284	5.3	1.5
Port/sherry	glass	90	20	1.8
Spirit	glass	35	40	1.4

What is your caffeine intake?

- 1 mug of instant coffee – 100 mg
- 1 cup of instant coffee – 75 mg
- 1 cup of brewed coffee – 100 mg
- 1 cup of black tea – 50 mg
- 1 cup of green tea – 10–50 mg
- 1 can of cola – 40 mg
- 1 can of 'energy' drink – up to 80 mg
- 50-g bar of dark chocolate – 40 mg
- 50-g bar of milk chocolate – 20 mg

Caffeine itself may even help reduce breast cancer risk. Two of three population studies have shown caffeinated (but not decaffeinated) coffee to reduce cancer risk. A 2006 study by Dr Baker and colleagues from the Department of Epidemiology in Buffalo in the USA, found that women drinking more than four cups of caffeinated coffee a day were 40 per cent less likely to get cancer than non-coffee drinkers.[14] Likewise, a 2006 study by Professor Narod at the Center for Research in Women's Health, Toronto, Canada, highlighted that women at high risk of breast cancer with the BRCA1 and BRCA2 genes, drinking at least four to six cups of coffee a day, were 25 to 70 per cent less likely to develop breast cancer.[15] Caffeine may help promote production of the less potent form of oestrogen (see page 38).

The benefits of caffeine on breast cancer risk may come as a surprise. Although caffeine is much maligned, none of the health fears surrounding caffeine have proved to be correct. Expert committees agree for most people there is no clear association between coffee consumption and the risk of increased blood pressure or heart disease.[16] However, for people with high blood pressure coffee and caffeine taken during stress might cause a slight increase in blood pressure. Neither is caffeine bad for the bones, provided there is an adequate intake of calcium. A 2003 review by researchers from the Bureau of Chemical Safety in Ottawa, Canada, concluded that mod-

What's in a cup of tea?

Tea comes from the leaves of the camellia sinesis plant, which is fermented to produce black tea or heated to give green tea. Black and green teas are both packed with health promoting antioxidant polyphenols (33 per cent of green tea; 3–10 per cent of black tea), but green tea is also the richest source of the flavonol epigallocatechin-3 gallate (EGCG) (approximately 100 milligrams per cup), which is evoking a great deal of interest as a possible agent for cancer prevention. As well as being a potent antioxidant EGCG enhances a cell's ability to repair its genetic material, blocks the sites in cells that attach potential cancer causing pollutants in chemicals or smoke, and also induces the death of cancer cells that have already begun to develop. The key question is how much green tea you would have to drink to see these effects in the body. The answer is we don't really know, but the best available evidence comes from a Japanese study, which showed protective effects from drinking ten small Japanese cups of green tea per day (equivalent to four to five standard UK cups). This dose should be safe, although pregnant women should be aware that green tea does contain 10 to 50 milligrams of caffeine per standard UK cup. Concerns that the anti-cancer properties of green tea affect many biochemical processes which are crucial in normal foetal development are not well founded. Recent animal studies have shown no adverse effects of EGCG in pregnant rats with doses equivalent to 200 milligrams per kilogram a day (up to one hundred cups of green tea a day).

erate daily caffeine intake at a dose level up to 400 milligrams a day (equivalent to 6 milligrams per kilogram of body weight a day) is not associated with adverse effects. Tea and coffee are diuretics, which mean they encourage the production of more urine and loss of water. It is therefore probably sensible to ensure only half of your drinks contain caffeine. Pregnant women should moderate their caffeine intake. Intakes in excess of 300 milligrams should be avoided since caffeine may increase risk of miscarriage or still birth.[17]

A range of decaffeinated teas and coffees is now widely available, which may be a personal preference to improve well-being and sleep patterns. These decaffeinated drinks are still packed with antioxidant flavonols and there are no obvious concerns with the chemicals used in the decaffeination process.

There is some evidence that green tea protects against breast cancer, although the effects are not thought to be as great as for cancers of the mouth, throat, stomach and bowel where ingested tea comes into direct contact with the cells. Black tea has no effect on breast cancer risk,[18] although drinking two to three cups of black tea a day appears to halve risk of heart disease.[19]

Summary

- *Each additional unit of alcohol (see page 79) consumed on a daily basis increases your risk of breast cancer by 7 per cent.*

- *A 250-ml glass of red wine on a daily basis (3½ units of alcohol) increases your risk of breast cancer by 25 per cent.*

- *Caffeine-containing drinks may help lower cancer risk, as they may promote production of a less potent form of oestrogen.*

- *Black and green teas are healthy drinks packed with antioxidant polyphenols.*

- *Green tea has many anti-cancer properties; four to five standard UK cups a day may help reduce cancer risk.*

Get your fats right

High fat diets have long been considered a major culprit in the current global epidemics of cancer, heart disease, obesity and diabetes. Fat is the most concentrated source of calories we eat, and weight for weight gives us twice as many calories as sugar or protein. Eating too much fat is fattening and bad for our health. Current guidelines suggest that women of healthy weight consume no more than 70–80 grams of fat per day (the equivalent of 10 to 12 teaspoons of fat), but you should obviously consume less if you are trying to lose weight! The main sources of fat in our diets are oils, butter, spreads, meat, dairy products and a lot are hidden fats found within pastry, cakes, biscuits and savoury snacks.

Fat is a crucial part of the diet, since fat is an essential nutrient that forms the building blocks of cells, nerves and many key hormones in the body. Critically, 1 to 2 grams each day of two particular fats, linolenic acid and linoleic acid fat, are essential for health. While some types of fat are clearly bad for the health, the important message for breast cancer (and indeed other diseases) is that it is the types of fat and the balance of these fats in the diet, not the overall fat intake that matters most.

The best evidence that cutting down all fat in the diet does not reduce cancer or heart disease risk comes from the 2006 Women's Health Initiative Study, which failed to show any significant reductions in rates of breast cancer, colorectal cancer or heart disease in women following a low fat diet (see page 84).

There are five main types of fat in the diet, namely saturated fats, monounsaturated fats, two types of polyunsaturated fats (omega-6 polyunsaturated and omega-3 polyunsaturated fats) and trans fats. Saturated, trans fats and omega-6 polyunsaturated fats all appear to increase breast cancer risk, while monounsaturated fats and omega-3 polyunsaturated fats seem to protect against breast cancer. The principal sources and effects of these fats are explained below.

Saturated fats and trans fats are usually solid at room temperature. Saturated fats are found in red meat, eggs and dairy products, such as butter, cheese and cream, also coconut oil and cocoa butter. Trans fats naturally occur in small amounts in meat, but the main source is foods containing naturally unsaturated fats that have been processed (hydrogenated) to become saturated, such as margarines, especially hard margarines, and processed biscuits, cakes, chips and crackers. This food process is a major health hazard.

Both saturated and trans fats are known to increase blood cholesterol levels, blood pressure and risk of heart disease, and have both been linked to risk of breast cancer. A recent UK study based on 13,000 women found women who ate more than 45 grams of

Low fat diets and breast cancer risk

The Women's Health Initiative (WHI) study is the only randomised trial of the effects of a low fat diet on breast cancer risk.

A group of 19,500 women were asked to reduce their total fat consumption and eat more fruit and vegetables. These women were then monitored over eight years during the 1990s and compared with another group of 29,300 women whose diet was unchanged.

On average the low fat diet group reduced fat intake by 20 grams a day and ate an additional portion of fruit or vegetables per day. There was a small reduction in breast cancer rates in the study group (9 per cent), which meant that 42 out of 10,000 women in the low fat group and 45 in the control group developed breast cancer each year. The researchers could not be sure that this small difference was not simply due to chance rather than an effect of the diet. Interestingly, women following the low fat diet did not lose weight.

The American researchers admit the difference between 'good' and 'bad' fats was not recognised when the study started. An approach that limits bad fats (saturated and trans fats) but encourages fats in nuts, fish and vegetable oils is more likely to have health benefits.

This study highlights two important points: first that a low fat diet per se does not help women to lose weight; second that reducing fat intake without controlling weight does nothing to protect us from cancer or heart disease.

saturated fat a day were twice as likely to get breast cancer as women eating less than 12 grams per day.[20] Likewise, women with high trans fat intakes (more than 3.6 grams a day) in a recent Dutch study had a third more breast cancer than women with minimal intakes.[21] These fats can promote the initiation and growth of cancer because they promote a host of harmful effects in our bodies, including the formation of damaging reactive free radical molecules, inflammatory factors, and higher levels of hormones such as insulin and oestrogen in the body. The advice leading on from this research is that you should have less than 7 per cent of your energy coming from saturated fat to limit your risk of breast cancer and you should try to eliminate trans fat from your diet. This matches current WHO guidelines to reduce risk of heart disease and diabetes.[22]

Beneficial monounsaturated fats are found in olive oil, rapeseed oil, olives, avocado, and nuts such as peanuts, almonds and hazelnuts. These fats are anti-inflammatory and are thought to be one of the main reasons that a Mediterranean diet is so good for the heart. Monounsaturated fat may also protect women against breast cancer. For example in the Dutch study mentioned above there were 40 per cent less cancers among women who ate at least 20 grams of monounsaturated fat per day.[21] Try to buy cold pressed or extra virgin olive oil wherever possible. These are more natural forms of the oil, which maintain higher levels of the potent antioxidant compounds (phenols) that may protect from cancer, than more processed heat and chemical treated forms. Women should aim to have 15 per cent of their energy from monounsaturated fat.

It has already been mentioned that there are two forms of polyunsaturated fats: omega-3 polyunsaturated fats found in oily fish, flaxseed, walnuts, rapeseed and soya oils, and omega-3 eggs (which are eggs from chickens fed high omega-3 diets); and omega-6 polyunsaturated fats found in vegetable oils such as sunflower, safflower and corn oil, chicken, turkey, and minimal amounts in white fish and shellfish. Both types of fat are good for the heart. These fats do, however, have vastly different effects on risk of cancer; numerous animal and breast cancer cell studies show that omega-6 types encourage breast cancer growth, while the anti-inflammatory omega-3 fats inhibit the promotion, progression and spread of breast cancer, and also of cancer of the bowel. Omega-3 fats may also help lower levels of oestrogen in menopausal women by blocking the enzyme aromatase (see page 37). You should aim to have no more than 6 per cent of your energy from omega-6 types and at least 2

per cent of your energy from omega-3 sources of fat. This trans-
lates as about 3 to 4 grams per day for omega-3 sources, ideally including fish since vegetable sources of these fats are not as readily used
by the body. You should aim to have four portions of oily fish a
week. If you do not eat fish consider taking a supplement, such as
one to two teaspoons of cod liver oil (2 grams of omega-3 fats) or
concentrated fish oil capsules providing 2 grams of omega-3 fats a
day. If you are strictly vegetarian you may wish to take one to two
teaspoons of flaxseed oil. Take care with this oil as it is unstable,
which means its health benefits are lost if it is heated.

It must be stressed that the right balance of fats in the diet is key.
Quite simply, you will not get the health benefits of omega-3 and
monounsaturated fat if you are still eating lots of saturated fat or
omega-6 fats in your diet. The main competition is between omega-
3 and the omega-6 fats. You can imagine your body as a machine
that processes both types of fat, but when omega-3 fats go through
the process, cancer inhibiting anti-inflammatory factors are produced, while if the omega-6 fats pass through the same machinery
very different cancer promoting factors result. If you consume lots
of omega-6 fat the omega-3 fats simply do not get a chance to enter
the machine so the beneficial effects do not occur. Experts recommend no more than three to four times as much omega-6 as omega-
3 fat be consumed. Our ancestors had a diet containing equal
amounts of these fats, while typically a Western diet contains ten
to 15 times as much omega-6 as it does omega-3 fat!

Summary

- *Low fat diets do not help reduce the risk of breast cancer or
  heart disease.*
- *The types of fats and the balance of fats in the diet is the
  important factor for health.*
- *Saturated, trans and omega-6 polyunsaturated fats all appear to
  increase breast cancer risk.*
- *Monounsaturated and omega-3 polyunsaturated fats seem to
  protect against breast cancer.*

Fruit, vegetables, beans and lentils

Everyone is being encouraged to eat more fruit and vegetables. The 'five a day' campaigns recommended the consumption of at least five portions of fruit and vegetables daily to protect against heart disease, help control blood pressure, maintain bone health and protect us against a number of cancers, including cancer of the bowel, lung, mouth and throat, larynx, oesophagus and stomach. The cancer protective effects of fruit and vegetables are hardly surprising since they are packed with vitamins (particularly vitamin C, the antioxidant carotenoids and folic acid) and phytochemicals (plant chemicals), which have a range of anti-cancer properties, acting as antioxidants, influencing hormone metabolism in the body, and directly exerting anti-cancer effects on tumour cells by blocking their ability to invade local tissues and develop their own blood supply, thus preventing the cells from becoming established. The protective effect of fruit and vegetables for cancers of the mouth and gut may be a result of the contact that the vegetables and fruits have with the tissues of the mouth and gut.

So does eating plenty of fruit and vegetables also ensure against breast cancer? Early studies showed quite convincing positive effects, however more recent, larger and more reliable studies have not shown this to be true. A recent overview of eight large, well-conducted international trials by researchers at Harvard School of Public Health in the USA suggested low intakes (one to two portions or less a day) may slightly increase risk, but there were no obvious benefits from higher intakes such as five a day or more.[23] Likewise, the largest study to date, the Europe-wide EPIC study based on 285,000 women, showed no difference in the likelihood of breast cancer whether women ate one or two portions per day or more than eight portions of fruit and vegetables a day.[24]

These studies do not however rule out specific breast cancer protection from particular types of fruit and vegetable. One of the most interesting groups of potential cancer protective vegetables are the cruciferous vegetables, such as broccoli, cabbage, Brussels sprouts, cauliflower, kale, pak choi, Chinese cabbage, turnip, kohlrabi, mustard and cress, watercress, radish and horseradish. These vegetables

The cancer protective and promoting fats in food

CANCER PROTECTIVE FATS
Sources

Monounsaturated fat	Omega-3 polyunsaturated fat
Olive oil	Salmon
Rapeseed (canola) oil	Sardines
Olive oil spreads	Mackerel
Avocados	Fresh tuna
Olives	Flaxseed
Peanuts/almonds	Walnuts
	Omega-3 enriched eggs

CANCER PROMOTING FATS
Sources

Omega-6 polyunsaturated fat	Saturated fat	Trans fat (hydrogenated)
Corn oil	Red meat, beef, lamb, pork, goose, duck	Hard margarines
Sunflower oil	Butter	Pies
Safflower oil	Full fat dairy products, eggs	Biscuits
Sesame oil	Margarines	Cakes, doughnuts, croissants
Chicken, turkey, game, i.e. rabbit, venison	Coconut	Fried snacks e.g. crisps
White fish	Meat products, e.g. sausages	
Shellfish, canned tuna	Chocolate	

Recommended amount of fat
for an average intake of 2000 calories a day

Fat	% energy	Amount in grams
Saturated	7	15
Trans	0	0
Omega-6 polyunsaturated fats	6	13
Omega-3 polyunsaturated fats	2	4
Monounsaturated	15	33

contain a number of key chemicals that are released when they are chewed or crushed. These chemicals (indole-3-carbinol and sulphorophane) promote the body's antioxidant enzyme defence, promote the production of a less potent form of oestrogen in the body (see page 38) and may directly inhibit cancer development by regulating the genetic repair gene, or by acting on developing cancer cells to prevent them becoming established and spreading within the tissues. Most studies have failed to link brassica intake specifically with risk reduction, although a recent study did find 20 to 40 per cent lower rates of breast cancer in women who regularly ate one to two portions of brassicas a day.[25] Scientists are aware that the relatively low activity of cancer fighting compounds in brassicas we eat may limit their effects. Current work at the John Innes Centre in Norwich, England, is breeding super broccoli, which has one hundred times more sulphorophane than the ordinary version. Other research is developing absorbable supplements, but the benefits of these approaches are far from proven. In the mean time, including brassicas in your diet is a possible, prudent anti-cancer measure.

Yellow and red fruit and vegetables and green leafy vegetables rich in the antioxidant carotenoids such as beta-carotene, beta-cryptoxanthin, lycopene and lutein may protect against breast cancer. Three studies, which looked at blood levels of carotenoids, have all found higher levels of consumption to be cancer protective.[26-28] The optimum intake is not known, but rich sources should be included in the diet. Rich sources of carotenoids are raw tomatoes and cooked/processed tomato products (from which lycopene is better absorbed), carrots, sweet potato, red and yellow peppers, pumpkin, beetroot, endive, grapefruit, mangoes, cantaloupe melon, peaches, nectarines, papaya, passion fruit, apricots, spinach, green peppers (capsicums), kale, lettuce, okra, Swiss chard, Brussels sprouts, cabbage, broccoli, sugar snap peas and asparagus (beta-carotene), squash (lutein), oranges, sweetcorn and orange juice (beta-cryptoxanthin). A report by the Nurses' Health Study in the USA suggests fruit and vegetables perhaps offer specific benefits only in women with a family history of cancer (see page 36).[29]

Fruit and vegetables should form part of any healthy eating plan, since they can help control your weight, being low in calories and a great way to fill up. Many women still have low intakes of fruits and in particular vegetables, which are the highest ranking cancer fighters. In fact, only 28 per cent of women in the UK manage five portions a day. Each additional serving of fruit or vegetables is estimated to cut your chances of heart disease by 4 per cent. The observation that each extra portion of fruit and vegetables significantly increases your life expectancy should be compelling enough reason to eat your greens, reds and yellows![30]

Polyphenols

The plant chemicals polyphenols are widespread in fruit and vegetables, cereals, pulses, spices and plant-derived drinks, such as tea, coffee, red wine and chocolate. Research into these fascinating compounds began in 1995; since then over 40,000 scientific papers have been published on cancer and polyphenols.

Polyphenols are important antioxidants in the body, mopping up harmful oxidising molecules and triggering cells to mobilise their own antioxidant defence mechanisms. It has already been explained how, for cancer to spread, the cancer cells need to become out of control, avoid dying and develop their own blood supply (see page 27). Studies in laboratories show polyphenols can limit each of these stages of tumour growth. How much of these polyphenols are actually absorbed and are able to reach where they are required in the body and their actual effect on cancer development is not known.

Current research efforts are attempting to improve the potency or availability of polyphenols. Since there are no obvious harmful effects from dietary intakes of polyphenols, advice in the mean time is to include these in the diet wherever possible. Key polyphenols currently being investigated, which are the most likely to have benefits for breast cancer protection, include resveraterol, found in grapes, wine, peanuts and peanut products; curcumin, found in the spice turmeric; quercetin, catechins and procyanids found in onions, apples, tea, broccoli, red wine, broad beans, lentils, apricots, berries, pears, dark chocolate, cocoa, cherries, figs, pomegranates and beetroot; gallates found in green tea (see page 81); and isoflavones found in pulses, beans and soya (although the beneficial effects of soya are far from certain – see page 113).

Lignans

Lignans are phytoestrogens – natural oestrogen-like substances found in plant foods. Lignans are not as similar to oestrogen as the phytoestrogens (in the form of isoflavones) in soya as they do not appear to have their oestrogen like or oestrogen blocking effects in the body (see page 113). The richest source of lignans is linseed (flaxseed), but they are also found in wholewheat and rye products, lentils, beans, seeds, cereals and many fruits, berries and vegetables. Lignans are absorbed and processed to their active forms (enterolactone and enterodiol) in the gut by naturally present bacteria. Enterolactone and enterodiol are important antioxidants, and also have the potential to halt the growth and spread of developing tumours. Despite these potential anti-cancer effects there is little evidence to suggest lignans prevent cancer. Only one of six studies has managed to find a protective effect for breast cancer, which was a modest 7 per cent reduction in risk for women with the highest blood levels of the active form enterolactone.[31]

Pulses and beans

Pulses and beans are packed with cancer protective polyphenols, fibre and lignans. A recent study showed that eating beans regularly (between two and four times a week) can reduce risk of breast

Nuts about nuts

Nuts were traditionally excluded from weight control diets due to their high fat content. Many nuts are great sources of potential cancer fighting nutrients, for instance, Brazil nuts are packed with selenium and peanuts with the anti-cancer polyphenol resveraterol. Many other nuts are great sources of anti-inflammatory omega-3 (walnuts) and monounsaturated fats (almonds, pecans, pistachios and peanuts), and all are known to reduce levels of fats in the blood and help protect against heart disease. Some researchers have speculated that nuts may even boost weight loss or help prevent weight gain, through exerting small increases in metabolic rate or by reducing absorption of energy from the diet. There is little to support these assertions, however the satiating power of nuts is likely to help with calorie and weight control.

cancer. A study from the Harvard School of Public Health tracked the diets of 90,000 nurses over eight years and found that women who ate beans at least twice a week had a 25 per cent lower risk of breast cancer than women who rarely ate them.[32]

Garlic
The allium vegetables onions, garlic, leeks, chives and shallots are a rich source of flavonols and the organosulphur compound diallyl disulfide. Animal and lab-based cell studies show convincing anti-cancer effects for these compounds. Garlic appears to confer some protection against colorectal and stomach cancer, but has no apparent influence on breast cancer risk.

Raw or cooked fruit and vegetables?
A question that is often asked is whether vegetables should be eaten raw or cooked for optimum protection. No studies have made a direct comparison of the cancer effects of raw versus cooked versions of the same vegetables. There is some evidence to suggest that raw veg-

etables may be better; boiling can leach out up to 60 per cent of the water soluble vitamins, such as vitamin C and folic acid, from vegetables. Likewise the enzyme that allows the body to obtain the cancer fighting chemicals from brassicas is destroyed by heating. Steaming broccoli dropped its isothiocyonate content by 60 per cent.[33] Microwaving has similar adverse effects, although cooking at a low power (< 540 w) for longer periods is the best way of retaining content.[34] However, cooking tomatoes increases the availability of lycopenes.

The nutritional content of fruit and vegetables varies hugely depending on growth and storage. Frozen fruit and vegetables may have slightly lower nutritional content than fresh due to blanching; however this content will still be higher than that found in older 'fresh' produce. Frozen and dried fruits and vegetables largely retain their phytochemical content and their antioxidant activity.

Summary

- *Fruit and vegetables reduce risk of cancers of the mouth and gut, and lung cancer, but do not appear to specifically influence breast cancer risk.*

- *Current research is focused on improving the potency and availability of specific breast cancer fighting chemicals in brassica vegetables, yellow and red fruit and vegetables, grapes, pulses, berries, pomegranates and beetroot – in the mean time it is prudent to include these in the diet whenever possible.*

- *Fruit and vegetables form an important part of any healthy eating plan to help control your weight and therefore lower your risk of breast cancer.*

- *Fruit and vegetables help reduce risk of heart disease.*

Low fat dairy products

A frequent concern among women wishing to limit their risk of breast cancer and of breast cancer patients is the possible adverse effects of dairy products. The researchers at Genesis do not believe that the benefits of milk free diets are supported by good scientific evidence; in fact some recent data suggest that dairy products, especially low fat versions, may actually help prevent the disease.

The belief that dairy foods may cause breast cancer was based on observations of high dairy intakes in Western women who have much higher rates of breast cancer than their Asian counterparts. There are many striking differences between Western and Asian women besides their dairy intakes. Higher weights, higher fat levels, high energy diets, lack of exercise, lower birth rates and a later age at first pregnancy can more than account for the higher rates of breast cancer in the West. Concerns that high levels of insulin-like growth factors and hormones (oestrogen and progesterone) in dairy products produced with modern intensive farming methods may promote breast cancer are largely unfounded. For example most insulin-like growth factor is broken down in the gut. The minimal amount absorbed is only a small proportion of the growth factor naturally present in the body. Recent data that dairy products are protective (outlined below) comes from the USA, where if anything milk has the highest levels of hormones and growth factors.

How can we be sure that the hormone and growth factors in milk are not an issue?

Modern farming methods mean that two-thirds of milk comes from pregnant cows, which increases the oestrogen and progesterone content somewhat. The concentrations of these hormones in milk are unlikely to pose a risk to our health, since the daily intake of hormones from milk is minute in comparison to the normal daily production of such hormones in women. They are certainly nowhere near the doses in oral contraceptives, which can contain 30 times the amounts found in milk.

High levels of growth hormone (insulin-like growth factor – IGF-1) occur in animals receiving bovine growth hormone. This controversial hormone is currently used in the USA, but was banned within the EU, Australia and New Zealand (as are imports produced with its use) in 1999 for animal welfare, health and political reasons. Dairy products within the EU, Australia and New Zealand consequently do not have high levels of IGF-1. Women can, however, still be reassured that where high dietary intakes of IGF-1 do occur they are unlikely to pose a cancer risk. IGF-1 is not as robust as oestrogen and progesterone, the majority of it is broken down in the stomach and will not be absorbed. There are limited data in humans but animal studies suggest ingested IGF-1 represented only 0.2 per cent of the amounts circulating in the body.[35]

Some dairy products are high in saturated fat and calories, such as full fat cheese, cream and butter, and should be avoided. However, a recent review on consumption of dairy products and breast cancer in the *American Journal of Clinical Nutrition* revealed four of the eight studies showed milk or dairy foods to reduce risk. The other four did not find a relationship, but, most importantly, none of these studies found milk to be harmful.[36] These studies suggest dairy products, in particular low fat dairy products such as skimmed and semi-skimmed milk, lower fat cheeses, such as cottage cheese, and low fat yoghurt, may actually protect women from developing breast cancer. Two large surveys from the USA, namely the Nurses' Health Study and the Cancer Prevention Study II Nutrition Cohort, show that drinking almost a pint of low fat milk or eating two portions of low fat dairy foods a day reduces your risk for breast cancer by 20 to 30 per cent.[37-39] What's more, there is also good evidence that dairy products help to protect against bowel cancer. Typically, drinking at least ½ pint of milk daily reduces risk by 20 per cent.[40]

The anti-cancer effects of low fat dairy foods are in fact not surprising. Dairy products are the major source of calcium and contain some vitamin D, which have well-known cancer protective effects. These nutrients work directly on cells to reduce growth and to inhibit their further development into cancerous cells. It is not clear whether non-dairy sources of calcium are as effective and calcium supplements do not seem to have these benefits, possibly as they are not as well absorbed as the calcium in milk (see page 96).

Vitamin D is found in oily fish, cereals, eggs and dried milk, but the body's store is largely determined by exposure to sunlight. Interestingly, greater exposure to sunlight seems to protect women

Intolerance to milk

Many people are unable to digest lactose in milk and are said to be lactose intolerant. An estimated 6 to 22 per cent of adults of Northern European, Caucasian descent are thought to be intolerant. Much higher rates are seen in people of Asian (up to 100 per cent of adults), and African (75 per cent of adults) and Hispanic (50 per cent of adults) descent. Many people discover that being lactose intolerant does not necessarily mean leaving dairy products out altogether and often find they can consume small amounts of lactose-containing foods (up to 1/3 pint/200 ml of milk a day), especially if taken with a meal. Foods such as cheese and live yoghurt are usually well tolerated, or you may prefer to use low lactose milks or utilise the commercially available lactose digestive aids.

from breast cancer, though these benefits must be balanced against the well-known risks of skin cancer from overexposure to the sun. A daily sunlight exposure of 20 minutes per day (without sunscreen since this inhibits vitamin D synthesis in the skin) and consumption of vitamin D-rich foods should meet requirements, although a supplement of 400 IU, 10 µg/day is recommended for those who are unable to achieve this. Calcium and vitamin D are also crucial for healthy bones, while calcium may help to control blood pressure and may even help to boost fat loss with a calorie controlled diet (see page 172).

Dairy products are also the main dietary source of the potential anti-cancer fat known as conjugated linoleic acid (CLA). This fat shows amazing anti-cancer effects on breast cancer cells and in animal studies, where it impedes growth and spread of cancer cells. The doses required for anti-cancer effects are at least three times greater then the usual dietary intake. Scientists are planning future studies with supplements, or naturally CLA enriched dairy products.[41]

Summary

- *Dairy products are a rich source of cancer fighting calcium and conjugated linoleic acid.*
- *Including two to three portions of dairy products a day in your diet reduces risk of breast cancer by 20 to 30 per cent.*
- *Vitamin D may help protect against breast and other cancers.*
- *Vitamin D requirements are met by a daily sunlight exposure of 20 minutes a day and eating vitamin D-rich foods, such as oily fish, cereals, eggs and dried skimmed milk.*

Whole grains and less refined starchy foods

Carbohydrates (sugars and starchy foods) are important sources of energy in the diet. The best types are wholegrain cereals, which have not been refined or processed and contain a whole list of potential cancer fighting nutrients, such as selenium, vitamin E, polyphenols and lignans. Many of these nutrients have antioxidant activity; weight for weight wholegrain breads or cereals have four to five times the antioxidant activity of vegetables![42]

Whole grains have been shown to be overall good for the health. Among a population of 40,000 post-menopausal women, those who ate one to three portions of whole grains per day had a greater life expectancy than women who ate just refined starchy foods. Over a nine-year follow up there were 25 per cent fewer deaths from cancer, heart disease and all other causes among women who ate whole grains. A further study from Sweden, the Malmö Diet and Cancer Study, showed that women who ate more than 25 grams of fibre per day were 36 per cent less likely to develop breast cancer.

Whole grains may help ensure the right balance of bacteria in the bowel, which keeps the bowel healthy and can help reduce re-absorption of oestrogen, thereby keeping down blood levels of the cancer promoter oestrogen (see page 38). A study showed that increasing fibre intake from 15 to 30 grams a day reduced oestrogen levels by 10 to 20 per cent.[43]

Glycaemic Index – what is it all about?

The latest trend in healthy and slimming diets is the low Glycaemic Index or GI diet. Some supermarkets are even labelling foods as high or low GI – so what does it all mean? Should we all be eating the low GI way?

Glycaemic index simply measures the impact a food has on blood sugar levels, that is how quickly starchy food is digested and enters the blood-stream. Foods that do not contain carbohydrates, such as meat and cheese, do not have a GI. High GI foods, such as white bread, break down quickly and raise blood sugars rapidly, while low GI foods break down slowly and gradually raise blood sugar. Glucose is absorbed directly into the blood-stream and is assigned the GI rank of 100. The GI of foods indicates how quickly blood sugar rises when a portion of the food containing 50 grams of carbohydrate is eaten.

Simply looking at lists of GI foods can be misleading. The actual impact of food on blood sugar depends on both the GI and the amount of carbohydrate it contains. This is known as the Glycaemic Load (GL). Some foods that have a high GI

Carbohydrates which have been refined or processed and the fibre removed, such as white bread and cakes and biscuits, are digested more quickly than whole grains and cause a rapid rise in blood sugar levels. This in turn causes a rapid rise in insulin in the blood-stream. Such foods are said to have a high 'glycaemic index' or GI. Pre-cancerous and cancer cell growth are fuelled by insulin and also glucose, which suggests these high GI foods could promote cancer growth. Few studies have shown clear links with the glycaemic load of the diet and breast cancer risk. Only two of the seven population studies that have examined this risk factor have shown any influence, and in these low GI foods were only protective among sedentary women.[44;] [45] There is some evidence that people following low GI diets are less likely to develop diabetes, high cholesterol and heart disease. Low (effect on blood sugar per 50 grams of carbohydrate) may be very low in carbohydrate, for example you might be concerned about eating watermelon, which has a GI of 72, but watermelon only has 5 grams of carbohydrate per portion. Remember that the GI of 72 applies to eating 1 kilogram of the fruit. A standard portion (100 grams) has a low glycaemic load of 4, and a minimal effect on blood sugar. A number of other healthy foods have a high GI, such as banana, potatoes, mango, wholemeal bread, couscous and broad beans, but there is no good evidence to suggest that these foods should be limited in the diet.

Not all low GI foods are healthy either. For example, chocolate and ice cream have a low GI and a diet based on these high fat foods is certainly not recommended.

A further confusion is that the GI of a food simply tells us the effect that a food has on blood sugar if it is eaten by itself. Few foods are eaten on their own and little is known of the effect that combining different foods has on the overall glycaemic load of a meal.

GI foods may be more satisfying and filling than high GI foods, which may help control food intake and weight. The large fluctuations in blood sugar experienced when eating refined carbohydrates are thought to increase appetite and carbohydrate cravings, making overeating more likely. Therefore, refined carbohydrates should be limited if you are trying to control your weight. To help you make the right choices, check out the table on page 100.

Many low GI foods are also wholegrain foods, which make it difficult to unravel the specific health benefits of GI from that of whole grain. A recent study linked four servings of wholegrains per day to a 40 per cent reduction in heart disease (which is equivalent to the benefits of a cholesterol lowering statin drug). In this study whole grain had a more powerful effect on health than the GI.[46] This

Healthy and refined carbohydrates

Healthy whole-grain carbohydrates	Refined carbohydrates
Wholemeal bread	White bread
Muesli, oats, bran or whole-wheat based cereals	Sugar-coated cereals, cornflakes, puffed rice cereals etc.
Whole-grain and rye crispbread	Crackers, cheese biscuits
Potatoes, boiled or baked with skins	Potato products, e.g. waffles, chips, mashed potato, crisps
Brown rice, wholewheat pasta and noodles, bulgur wheat, couscous	White rice and pasta, pastry, pizza bases
	Cakes, biscuits, sugar

is not surprising as wholegrain foods also contain many health giving vitamins and chemicals. The science behind low GI diets is limited but the benefits of wholegrain foods have been known for many years. The best advice is to go for wholegrain and the GI will, on the whole, look after itself.

Summary

- *Eating wholegrain rather than refined processed starchy foods may reduce breast cancer risk by 30 per cent.*
- *Wholegrain cereals contain many potential cancer fighting nutrients such as selenium, vitamin E, polyphenols and lignans.*
- *Whole grains maintain the right balance of bacteria in the bowel, which controls blood levels of the cancer promoter oestrogen.*
- *Refined or processed starchy foods cause rapid rises in blood sugar levels, and have been linked to heart disease and diabetes.*
- *Wholegrain foods help regulate blood sugar levels, which may help with weight control.*

Meat, poultry, fish and eggs

As already discussed, meat, poultry, fish and eggs contain different types of fat, which may have different impacts on breast cancer risk. Red meat (lamb, pork, beef) and eggs are a source of saturated fats, while chicken and turkey contain some saturated and some polyunsaturated fat, which in large enough quantities may promote breast cancer. This does not mean excluding meat, poultry and eggs totally from the diet; many lean cuts of meat and poultry with the skin removed can safely be included and eggs are relatively low in fat, so up to six eggs a week is fine, indeed you may even wish to include omega-3 enriched eggs. Fish and seafood, especially oily fish, are the richest sources of the anti-inflammatory cancer protective omega-3 unsaturated fats, and are an important part of a healthy diet. It is important to get the right balance of fish and meat in the diet. Recent evidence suggests the potential cancer protective effects of eating more fish will not occur alongside a high meat or poultry intake. A recent population study in 35,298 Singapore Chinese women found women eating at least three portions of oily fish week were 30 per cent less likely to get breast cancer. Women were at highest risk, almost twice as likely to get breast cancer, if they had a low intake of fish and a high intake of chicken and meat.[47]

Three-quarters of salmon bought in the UK is now farmed and the nutrient content of farmed compared to natural wild (expensive, restricted availability) versions has been under close scrutiny. Farmed fish certainly has a higher fat content, providing 10 to 14 grams per portion rather than 5 to 9 grams per portion. It still provides a good source of the omega-3 fats, but just a bit more of the omega-6. The overall balance of these fats is crucial but will depend on the rest of your diet. Canned fish such as salmon, sardines, mackerel and pilchards are the best source of omega-3 fats as is fresh, but not canned tuna, as the canning process removes its beneficial oils.

A frequent concern is the potential harmful effects of consuming the toxins (dioxins, PCBs and mercury) found in fish, especially oily fish, which can then accumulate in the body. The UK Food Standards Agency recently acknowledged the presence of toxins in fish in its expert report 'Advice on fish consumption benefits and risk', but concluded that the health benefits of fish outweighed the potential harm of these low doses of toxins.[48] The main concern is the possible adverse effects of toxins on unborn children. Shark, marlin and swordfish are especially high in mercury. Herrings/kippers have the highest dose of dioxins and PCB, mackerel and salmon have intermediate levels, white fish and trout have the lowest amounts. Women who are already pregnant or who are planning to become so can safely include up to two portions of oily fish per week and unlimited amounts of white fish, but should avoid shark, marlin and swordfish. For the general population, a minimum of one to two portions of oily fish a week is recommended to protect our hearts but no more than four portions per week, including no more than two portions of herring or kipper.

The way meat and fish is cooked may also impact on cancer risk. When meat, chicken and fish are cooked at high temperatures they form potential cancer causing chemicals known as heterocyclic amines and polycyclic aromatic hydrocarbons (PAHs). Fewer heterocylic amines are produced when food is stewed, braised or microwaved, slightly higher levels are seen when deep fried or roasted, but the highest levels, often tenfold greater, are seen when food is pan fried, barbecued or grilled, especially when it is well done, charred or burnt! Marinating meat with vinegar and lemon juice helps prevent the formation of heterocylic amines. These substances are formed from a reaction in meat protein and are not related to fat content; some of the highest levels are seen in chicken. A minority of women (3 per cent) have genes that convert heterocyclic amines to their active cancer causing forms; if these women eat lots of well-cooked meats cooked at high temperatures they are six times as likely to develop breast cancer.[49] Well-done meats pose a low or negligible breast cancer risk for most women, but are bad news for risk of bowel cancer, as is too much of any red meat.

Smoked, cured and processed meats are high in polycyclic aromatic hydrocarbons and also high in nitrites, which can produce cancer causing nitrosamines in the body. These foods have not been specifically linked to breast cancer but do increase risk of bowel and stomach cancer.

The recommendation to achieve the optimum balance of meat and fish in your diet is to try to include two to four portions of oily fish a week; limit lean red meat to no more than four times a week; the remaining meals should be an equal balance of fish and poultry with ideally a pulse based/vegetable meal two to four times a week.

Summary

- *Omega-3 fats found in oily fish may help protect against breast cancer.*
- *The potential cancer protective effects of eating more fish will not occur alongside a high meat or poultry intake – you need the right balance of fish and meat.*
- *Oily fish contain small amounts of dioxins, PCBs and mercury; eating fewer than four portions of oily fish per week ensures these do not accumulate to toxic levels in the body.*
- *Cancer causing chemicals form in overcooked or charred meat, chicken and fish, which can promote breast cancer in approximately 3 per cent of women.*
- *Smoked cured meats increase risk of stomach and bowel cancer but not breast cancer.*

Processed food and salt

Many people regularly eat processed food and ready meals. There is no obvious cancer risk from food additives and arcylamide, a potential cancer causing chemical, which forms naturally in baked or fried foods (see page 104). Processed foods are not part of your Genesis Breast Cancer Prevention Diet, however, as they are too high in salt and fats, particularly the unhealthy saturated and hydrogenated fats, which increase breast cancer risk. Salt is not specifically linked to breast cancer, but is linked to cancer of the stomach, and high blood pressure. High blood pressure makes you three times more likely to have a stroke or develop heart disease later in life. Too much salt encourages loss of calcium from the bones and

What is arcylamide?

Arcylamide is a cancer causing chemical that forms naturally in foods that are baked or fried, but not boiled. Main dietary sources include crisps, French fries, crisp breads, crackers, coffee, cereals and meatballs. Evidence from animal and risk assessment models suggests that risk for cancer in those exposed to more than 1 µg/kg per day may only be 1.006 to 1.05 per cent. Only 1 to 2 per cent of women in a recent survey had an intake in excess of this. A recent population study among 43,000 women in Sweden failed to link arcylamide intake to breast cancer risk and current evidence suggests there is no significant public health risk of breast cancer associated with dietary intake of arcylamide.[50]

the risk of thinner bones and osteoporosis. You should have no more than 6 grams of salt a day; on average people are actually having about 9.5 grams of salt a day, which is nearly 60 per cent more salt than is recommended as a maximum!

Three-quarters of the salt content of the average diet is found within processed foods, such as ready meals, soups, sauces, biscuits and breakfast cereals, not shaken on food or the pinch added when cooking. One ready meal for example can contain 6 grams of salt, the maximum recommended intake in one go! Salt is also called sodium chloride. If sodium is listed in the nutritional information you can work out how much salt it contains by multiplying the sodium by 2.5. So if a portion of food contains 1.2 grams of sodium, then it contains about 3 grams of salt. Look at the salt content in some familiar processed foods set out in the table opposite.

Not all processed foods are bad; some foods such as breakfast cereals are fortified with beneficial vitamins, such as folic acid and B vitamins. Tomato-based products such as sauces, soup and baked beans may be high in salt but they are also a key source of cancer protective lycopene in the diet.

Additives

Many people suspect that the chemical additives in food are cancer causing. This is extremely unlikely since each of the additives or E numbers (as they are called in the EU) listed on packaged foods have passed rigorous safety tests to ensure they do not damage genetic material, and cause cancer in animal models at much higher doses than humans would ever consume. This approval is constantly monitored, reviewed and amended in the light of new scientific data, as sometimes additives once considered safe have later been found to be dangerous, such as the azo dyes that were once used in butter.

Any chemical undergoes intense scrutiny before it is allowed to be added to foods. This is in contrast to natural substances such as vitamins and minerals, which until recently were not subject to any regulations or safety testing. An EU directive (of August 2005) now means only vitamins and minerals that have been proven to be safe are permitted in food supplements. This directive has banned the inclusion of some minerals that were previously allowed in food supplements (tin, silicon, boron, cobalt and vanadium).

Some of the most common additives include the antioxidant E300, which is vitamin C and curcumin (E100), a yellow colour extracted from turmeric roots. There are downsides to additives as there are possible links between artificial food colours and

Salt content of processed foods

Food	Salt content – grams
Bag of crisps (40 g)	1.2
Pizza (7 inch)	1.5
Sliced bread (4 slices)	1.8
Canned soup (½ can)	2.5
Quarterpounder and French fries	3.6
Takeaway Chinese meal (1 portion)	5
Instant noodle snack	10

preservatives and children's behaviour, and the potential that com-
binations of additives taken when a mixture of processed food is
eaten may have different effects.

Sweeteners

Artificial sweeteners such as saccharin and aspartame, acesulphame-
K and alitame are often under suspicion of causing cancer, but there
is little evidence to back these claims. Saccharin has been used in
diet products for over 50 years. Since 1981, foods containing saccharin carry a warning label that high doses of saccharin fed to rats
induced the development of bladder cancer. It is interesting to note
that feeding vitamin C in similar doses also causes cancer!

Aspartame entered the market in 1981, and has not been linked
to cancer in either animal or population studies. One study suggested
a slight increase in bladder cancer among heavy users of any artificial sweetener (>1700 mg/day, more than ten cans of diet drink a
day). The newer generation sweeteners such as acesulphame-K, alitame, sucralose and neotame do not have obvious cancer causing
or gene toxicity. They have not been in use long enough for their
effects to be studied in populations. Current evidence suggests sweeteners are safe and have a negligible effect on cancer risk.[51]

Summary

- *Processed foods are often high in salt.*
- *Salt is not specifically linked to breast cancer, but it is linked to cancer of the stomach and high blood pressure.*
- *Arcylamide is a cancer causing chemical, which forms naturally in baked or fried foods. There is no evidence that breast cancer is linked to levels of arcylamide found in the diet.*
- *Food additives undergo rigorous safety testing before they are permitted in foods and have not been linked to cancer risk.*
- *Artificial sweeteners are safe to include in the diet and have not been linked to cancer risk.*

What about nutritional supplements?

An estimated 20 to 30 per cent of adults in Western countries regularly take nutritional supplements. For many trying to reduce their risk of cancer the quest for a quick fix nutritional supplement to stave off the disease is an appealing prospect. Despite the popularity of supplements, there is surprisingly little data to support them as a means of prevention; some supplements may even put you at higher risk.

Being deficient in nutrients such as vitamin C, selenium, vitamins E and A, vitamin D and calcium increases cancer risk. None of the studies have however shown that large doses of these nutrients in excess of your requirement further lower risk.[52] The recent French Su Vi Max study (13,000 French men and women) found men taking a daily antioxidant and mineral supplement (120 mg vitamin C, 30 mg vitamin E, 6 mg beta-carotene,100 mg selenium, 20 mg zinc) over seven-and-a-half years were 30 per cent less likely to develop cancer, but it did not have any effect on the chances of a woman developing breast or indeed any other type of cancer as the women in the study were already meeting their requirements from their diets.[53]

Previous efforts to prevent other cancers with supplements have actually done more harm than good. Two large studies designed to prevent lung cancer with beta-carotene in smokers and those exposed to asbestos, actually showed an increase in risk. The US-based Beta-carotene and Vitamin A Efficacy Trial (CARET) was stopped early because of clear evidence of harm; there were 28 per cent more lung cancers and 17 per cent more deaths in those taking the supplements. Likewise, in the Finnish Alpha-Tocopherol Beta-Carotene (ATBC) Cancer Prevention Study, beta-carotene increased cancer of the lung and also cancer of the prostate and stomach.[54] A recent Cochrane overview, which reviews the most high-quality, up-to-date research, reported attempts to prevent cancers of the oesophagus, stomach, bowel, liver and pancreas with antioxidants actually found combined beta-carotene and vitamin A, and vitamin E supplements, increase rates by as much as a third; if the findings of this study are correct it suggests that one out of every 100 users of such supplements may die prematurely from taking them,[55] probably as high doses of antioxidants can actually start to behave as oxidants, paradoxically increasing oxidation.

There is some evidence that selenium supplements (200 µg) may be cancer protective, at least for cancer of the prostate, lung and colon, but not specifically for breast cancer. Selenium is a key factor in the antioxidant defence system, and also helps to repair genetic material, and impedes the growth and development of cancer cells. A dose of 1 mg per kilogram of body weight per day is required to maximise antioxidant activity in the body, which can be met from the diet or from low dose supplements (see box opposite). The optimum dose for the anti-cancer effects is thought to be considerably higher, but supplements are not currently recommended for this purpose. There remain questions over whether the form of selenium in the majority of supplements (selenium methionine) is truly beneficial, while high doses of supplements (over 400 µg) are not advised as they can be toxic and damage nails, hair and nerves and lead to gut problems.

Vitamin C is an antioxidant, which also has important roles in making connective tissue and nerves in the body. Vitamin C probably has more health claims linked to it than almost any other nutrient. Its most enthusiastic advocate was Linus Pauling (Nobel prize winner for chemistry in 1954), whose book *Vitamin C, the Common Cold and Flu* was first published in 1976. Since then vitamin C has been claimed to protect against cancer, heart disease, cataracts, diabetes, asthma, arthritis, Parkinson's disease, autism and depression. There is no reliable evidence to support these claims; no studies have shown vitamin C to protect against any of these diseases, including cancer. Doses of vitamin C of more than 1 gram a day may actually be bad for the health, can cause abdominal pain and diarrhoea, and may increase risk of kidney stones. Of concern for those trying to protect themselves from cancer, vitamin C actually becomes a pro-oxidant at these higher levels, which has been shown to damage the genetic material in cells and this could actually promote cancer.[56] The vitamin C story is a salutary lesson. Linus Pauling was a great chemist and had the idea that high doses of vitamin C were important, but did not do the appropriate studies on humans to prove his idea was correct. Just having an idea,

What about selenium?

Selenium is present in the soil and enters the food chain through plants. Soil levels and therefore dietary intake is high in the USA but is poor in the UK, much of Europe and New Zealand. There has been a substantial fall in selenium intake in the UK in the past 20 years due to reductions in selenium-rich wheat imports from the USA. On average intake in the UK is only half of the recommended intake, which may increase susceptibility to heart disease, asthma and infections. The best dietary sources of selenium are Brazil nuts and offal; the table below details further sources. If you are unable to meet your intake from foods, you may consider supplementing your diet with a 50-µg selenite or selenium methionine supplement.

Food	Selenium content µg	% of daily selenium requirement
Brazil nuts (25 g)	64	100
Kidney (100 g)	145	240
Liver (100 g)	42	70
Fish (150 g)	24	40
Fruit and vegetables (600 g)	12	20
Milk (600 ml)	9	15
Beef (100 g)	8	13
Cereals (50 g)	7	11
Bread (3 slices)	4.5	8

however illustrious you are, does not prove something is right – you have to test to see if it is true.

The clear message from these studies is that simply adding a vita-min/mineral supplement to your diet is unlikely to reduce cancer risk.

Recommended vitamin and mineral intakes (UK)

	Minimum safe intake	Maximum safe intake
Vitamin A	700 μg	> 1.5 mg can increase risk of fractures
Beta-carotene	800 μg	20 mg caused lung cancer in smokers
Vitamin D	10 μg or 400 IU*	< 50 μg or 2000 IU
Vitamin E	4 mg	> 50 mg may increase risk of stroke and heart disease
Vitamin K	70 μg	Not toxic
Thiamine (B1)	0.9 mg	Not toxic
Riboflavin (B2)	1.3 mg	Not toxic
Nicotinamide	16 mg	Not toxic
Pyridoxidine (B6)	1.4 mg	> 10 mg leads to nerve damage/memory loss
Folic acid	400 μg	< 1000 μg as may mask vitamin B12 deficiency if present
Vitamin B12	1.5 μg	Not toxic
Biotin	10–200 μg	Not toxic
Pantothenic acid	3–7 mg	Not toxic
Vitamin C	200 mg	> 1 g/day can cause diarrhoea and may damage genetic material
Calcium	700 mg	>2000 mg/day may interfere with absorption of other minerals such as iron
Magnesium	300 mg	Not toxic
Boron		5 mg/day disturbs reproductive cycle, increases oestrogen levels in middle-aged and older women
Chromium	> 25 μg	> 10,000 μg impairs reproduction
Copper	1.2 mg	> 5 mg has effects on the gut and is toxic to the liver

Recommended vitamin and mineral intakes (cont)

	Minimum safe intake	*Maximum safe intake*
Iodine	140 µg	Not toxic
Iron	8.7 mg	› 17 mg may lead to free radical damage and cancer
Selenium	60–75 µg	› 400 µg may lead to selenium toxicity and oxidative stress; affects hair, nails, gut, nerves and balance
Zinc	9.5 mg	› 25 mg reduces iron and copper absorption

* Recommended for pregnant or breastfeeding women, housebound, people of Asian origin, or if you always cover up all your skin when you're outside.

Concentrating on whole foods (such as whole grains, low fat dairy products, fruit and vegetables) is a far more effective way of keeping healthy. To sum up, it is better to get your nutrients from foods rather than supplements!

However, as previously mentioned it may be prudent for regular modest drinkers to include a daily 400-µg folic acid supplement to reduce their cancer risk (see page 78). This dose of folic acid is also recommended for all women planning to conceive to reduce the risk of neural tube defects in their babies. In the USA and Canada all flour products are fortified with folic acid. Voluntary fortification of certain foods, mainly breakfast cereals, occurs in the UK, Australia and New Zealand, and may help boost your levels.

Vitamin D and calcium help maintain bone health, reducing risk of osteoporosis. For most people exposure to sunlight will be more effective than supplements to boost vitamin D stores. If you are housebound, of Asian origin or always cover up all your skin when you're outside you will benefit from taking a daily supplement of vitamin D, 400 IU per day and calcium, 700 mg.

The recommended and safe limits for vitamin and mineral intakes are shown in the table opposite, notably care should be taken with

Other minerals

Zinc is a key nutrient that has an important role in the immune system, wound healing and bone health, and is a key factor in the main antioxidant enzymes. Most people do not need a zinc supplement; good food sources of zinc include meat, shellfish, milk and dairy foods, wholegrain bread and cereal products.

Magnesium is a key nutrient that is important for healthy bones and controlling blood pressure. It is also pivotal for achieving optimal control of blood sugar levels, by helping to ensure the effective action of insulin in the body. You should not need to take a magnesium supplement. Instead eat plenty of whole grains and fresh fruit and vegetables.

high doses of zinc since this can damage DNA, the first key step in the cancer process, and boron (now banned in supplements in the EU), which can increase levels of oestrogen in middle-aged and older women.

Summary

- *It is important to meet your requirements for vitamin C, selenium, vitamins E and A, vitamin D and calcium. Large doses of these nutrients in excess of your requirements, however, do not lower your cancer risk.*

- *Beta-carotene supplements increase risk of cancer of the lung, prostate and stomach in smokers.*

- *Selenium supplements (200 μg) may protect against cancer of the prostate, lung and colon, but not specifically breast cancer.*

- *High doses of vitamin C over 1 gram per day may damage genes in cells, which could actually promote cancer.*

- *Modest drinkers should include a daily 400-μg folic acid supplement to reduce their breast cancer risk.*

Soya foods

The idea that soya foods (tofu, soya milk, textured vegetable protein, miso) may protect against breast cancer is a popular health claim. The team at Genesis believe that the jury is still out on soya – surprisingly there is little evidence that eating soya as an adult reduces breast cancer risk and equally there is insufficient evidence of its harms, so on balance the team at Genesis feel it is safe to include soya as part of a healthy, balanced diet.

The case for soya on paper is certainly compelling and came originally from the striking observation of much higher soya consumption of Asian women who have much lower rates of breast cancer than Western women. Soya foods are the major source of amazing oestrogen-like substances called isoflavones. The two main isoflavones in soya are dazdein and genestein, which are structurally very similar to oestrogen. Oestrogen affects the growth and development of a number of tissues in the body including breast cells, by fitting into an oestrogen shaped lock (or receptor) on the cells, which triggers the cells to grow and develop. Isoflavones can fit in the lock, and block oestrogen from binding to the cell, preventing oestrogen driven cell growth. Isoflavones have other potential anti-cancer effects including acting as an antioxidant, inhibiting tumour growth and progression. Isoflavones can lower a woman's natural levels of oestrogen and also promote oestrogen to be metabolised to the less harmful (2-hydroxysterone) form rather than the cancer causing (16-hydroxysterone) form (see page 38). Isoflavones we eat need to be processed by bacteria in the bowel to their active forms, and only one out of three can achieve this process.

If soya is consumed before or at the time of puberty it is thought to encourage breast cells to undergo changes similar to those which occur during pregnancy, which, as described earlier, makes the cells more resistant to damage and cancer development later in life.[57] Many studies have shown that eating soya during adolescence protects against the later development of breast cancer. For example, a study of 1459 breast cancer cases and 1556 age-matched healthy women in the Shanghai Breast Cancer Study showed that women who consumed at least 11 grams of soya protein a day (at least

½ pint/300 ml of soya milk) during adolescence were half as likely to develop breast cancer in later life than those who didn't eat any at all.[58]

So far so good, but there are also some worrying aspects of soya – which may, in some situations, help to promote breast cancer. The Committee on Toxicity of Chemicals in Food and Consumer Products and the Environment recently highlighted concerns that as well as blocking oestrogen, soya foods can also have oestrogen-like effects on the breast.[59] This is supported by two studies including work by Professor Bundred and a further study by scientists at the University of California, who found high soya diets (typically 1 to 1½ pints of soya milk or 100 grams of tofu/TVP) actually stimulated breast cells to multiply,[60;61] which may increase their cancer potential.

So what is the balance of these good and bad effects? Earlier reports from small studies showed soya to be protective. Seven of the nine more recent larger population studies in Western and Japanese women failed to link soya intake with risk. One UK-based study found rates of breast cancer were 20 to 40 per cent higher among women with the highest blood levels of soya isoflavones.[62]

Soya during childhood or adolescence may be beneficial, but current evidence does not recommend increasing soya intake as an adult to minimise your breast cancer risk. Moderate amounts of soya foods can safely be included as part of a healthy diet. However, high soya intakes may be an issue in women with low levels of oestrogen, such as post-menopausal women, or in breast cancer patients taking tamoxifen or anastrazole (see page 144).

If soya foods were really so harmful you would not expect to see the low rates of breast cancer among the Japanese and Chinese where women typically have ten times the amount of soya foods as in the UK, typically 3 to 4 ounces/90 to 115 grams of tofu a day. This suggests it is safe to include soya in the diet, provided that the other essential components of their lifestyle are met, in other words if it is part of an energy restricted, healthy lifestyle. Current evidence suggests soya foods have a neutral effect on risk, so if you enjoy soya products, it seems reasonable to continue to use them. They should not, for example, be chosen in preference to foods that are known to be protective, so don't choose soya milk in preference to low fat dairy milk. On the other hand, a soya meat substitute is a much better choice than a high animal fat meat, which may increase risk. Soya foods are good low fat sources of protein, which are well known to reduce cholesterol levels.

As well as soya foods there is growing interest in the effects of isolated phytoestrogen in a tablet form. The effect of these supplements on breast cancer and health is not known. A recent study looked at the effect of red clover supplements (which are isoflavones) on the density of breasts, which is a measure of gland tissue and risk. One year of supplements did not affect density and is therefore presumed not to affect risk.[63] These supplements are not currently recommended, as they are not especially helpful for controlling hot flushes, and they are not as effective as soya foods in lowering cholesterol. These tablets are especially not recommended for breast cancer patients receiving anti-hormone therapy (see page 143).

Summary

- *Soya contains phytoestrogens, which have a large number of potential anti-cancer properties.*

- *Soya intake during adolescence may protect women from developing breast cancer later in life.*

- *The risks/benefits of starting to eat soya as an adult on breast cancer risk are not known.*

- *Soya foods can help to lower cholesterol.*

- *Isolated phytoestrogen supplements do not seem to have the same effects as soya foods and are not recommended.*

Vegetarian and vegan diets

There is no evidence that vegetarians or vegans have less cancer or indeed other diseases than those who include meat, fish and dairy products, fruit and pulses as part of a healthy balanced diet. The choice to be vegetarian or vegan should be based on ethical rather than health grounds.

Vegetarians and vegans need to optimise their intake of key cancer protective nutrients found in animal products. For those who do not eat fish, it is important to include plenty of vegetable sources of beneficial omega-3 fats as found in flaxseed, pumpkin seeds, walnuts and rapeseed (canola) oil. Meat, fish and nuts are the best sources of selenium in the diet so strict vegetarians should ensure they are eating enough nuts, especially Brazil nuts, so try to eat a couple every day.

You have already seen evidence that calcium-rich diets may be cancer protective. It can be difficult to achieve these cancer protective calcium intakes from vegetable sources alone, so you should consider 700-mg calcium supplementation, although current evidence questions whether calcium supplements are as cancer protective as calcium acquired from dairy products.

It is important to secure a good intake of iron; good vegetarian sources include pulses, green vegetables such as watercress, broccoli, spring greens and okra, bread and fortified breakfast cereals. It is easier to absorb iron from these foods if they are eaten with foods that contain vitamin C, so have some fruit or vegetables, or a glass of fruit juice with your meal. Avoid drinking tea or coffee with your meals because these make it harder for the body to absorb iron. It's best to wait at least half-an-hour after eating before having a cuppa. Vitamin B12 is not naturally found in the vegan diet, so vegans should include yeast extract, fortified bread, fortified breakfast cereals or take a daily 2-µg supplement.

Summary

- *Vegetarians and vegans do not have less cancer than those who include meat, fish and dairy products as part of a healthy balanced diet.*

- *Vegetarians need to ensure an adequate intake of omega-3 fats, selenium and iron.*

- *Vegans need to ensure an adequate intake of omega-3 fats, selenium, iron, calcium, vitamin D and vitamin B12.*

Tips for keeping your bones healthy

As many as one in three women are at risk of developing osteoporosis. There are, however, several ways in which you can help reduce the rate of thinning in your bones:

- Include calcium-rich foods (aim for an intake of 700 mg per day) such as low fat dairy products, green leafy vegetables and bony fish in your diet.
- Have regular exposure to at least 15 to 20 minutes of daylight each day and include dietary sources of vitamin D (oily fish, eggs, dried milk) to ensure adequate vitamin D stores (see page 111).
- Limit your intake of salt and alcohol, as these reduce the body's ability to absorb and retain calcium.
- Do not smoke, as this blocks bone building cells.
- Plenty of fruit and vegetables lowers acid load in the body, which helps preserve bone (nine portions per day).
- Take regular weight-bearing exercise, i.e. aerobics, brisk walking, tennis and weight training.
- Fizzy drinks and caffeine can increase loss of calcium from the body and lead to bone thinning. Current research shows it is safe to include these foods in your diet provided you ensure that you have a good calcium intake.

Food	Calcium – mg
200 ml pint milk, semi-skimmed/skimmed	235
Cheese, low fat hard/Edam	270
Low fat yoghurt, 150 g	225
Fromage frais, 150 g	135
Canned sardines, 100 g	500
Canned pilchards, 100 g	300
Spinach/curly kale, steamed, 100 g	150
Watercress, 100 g	170
Tofu, steamed, 100 g	510

'How healthy is my diet?'
Genesis healthy diet ready reckoner

What you eat and drink has an impact on your risk of breast cancer, your weight and your general health. Fill in the following quiz to find out how healthy your diet is:

Fruit, vegetables, pulses and beans

How often do you eat fresh fruit?	____ portions/day
How often do you eat fresh or frozen vegetables?	____ portions/day
How often do you eat beans, pulses or lentils?	____ portions/week ____ never

Carbohydrates (starchy foods)

What type of bread do you regularly eat?	____ White bread/brown bread ____ Wholemeal, rye, bread
Which breakfast cereals do you regularly eat?	____ Porridge, bran cereals, wholewheat cereals, sugar free muesli ____ Cornflakes, puffed rice, sugar coated or crunchy cereals, sweetened muesli, instant oats
What type of pasta/rice do you use?	____ White ____ Wholewheat/brown
Do you eat bulgur wheat/couscous/quinoa?	____ portions/week
How often do you eat cakes/biscuits?	____ portions/week
How often do you eat pastry/puddings?	____ portions/week
How often do you eat sweets/chocolates?	____ portions/week

Protein foods

How often do you eat beef, lamb or pork?	____ portions/week
How often do you eat processed meat or meat products, i.e. bacon, salami, sausages, beef burgers, pâté?	____ portions/week
How often do you eat chicken or turkey?	____ portions/week
How often do you eat game i.e. venison?	____ portions/week
How often do you eat oily fish, i.e. fresh tuna, trout, canned or fresh salmon, mackerel?	____ portions/week

How often do you eat white fish, i.e. cod, haddock, plaice?	____ portions/week
How often do you eat seafood, i.e. prawns, mussels?	____ portions/week
How often do you eat soya products, i.e. tofu?	____ portions/week
How often do you eat nuts and seeds	____ portions/week

Fats

What type of cooking oil do you use?	____ Olive/rapeseed (canola)/ nut oils ____ Sunflower/corn oil ____ Lard/butter
What type of spread do you use?	____ Olive oil spread/ soya margarine ____ Sunflower margarine ____ Butter ____ Low fat spread
How often do you eat crisps/ savoury snack biscuits?	____ portions/week
How often do you eat shop bought biscuits/cakes?	____ portions/week
How often do you eat shop bought pastry/puddings?	____ portions/week
How often do you eat chocolate?	____ portions/week

Dairy products

What type of milk do you drink?	____ None ____ Full fat cows' milk Semi-skimmed or skimmed ____ cows' milk Sheep or ____ goats' milk
Do you eat cheese?	____ None ____ 0–4 oz (110 g) per week More than 4 oz ____ (110 g) per week
How often do you eat cottage cheese?	____ portions/week
Do you ever you eat low fat yoghurt or fromage frais?	____ None ____ portions/week
How often do you eat full fat yoghurt, i.e. Greek style?	____ portions/week

How often do you eat cream?	____ portions/ week
How often do you eat ice cream?	____ portions/week

Drinks

How many drinks (non-alcoholic) do you have each day?	____
How many alcoholic drinks do you have each week?	____ Glasses of wine ____ Spirits ____ Beer
How often do you drink fizzy drinks?	____ Regular drinks/week ____ Diet drinks/week
How often do you drink fruit juice?	____ Glass/day

Salt

Do you add salt to your food?	____ Yes ____ No
How often do you eat ready meals or processed food?	____ portions/week
How often do you have takeaway meals like burgers, Indian or Chinese meals?	____ times/week
How often do you have salty snacks, i.e. crisps, savoury biscuits	____ portions/week

Genesis healthy diet ready reckoner scoring sheet

Compare your answers to the recommended intakes below to score your diet...

Fruit, vegetables, pulses and beans	*Score*
Fresh fruit	1 for each portion/day
Fresh or frozen vegetables	1 for each portion/day
Beans, pulses or lentils	1 for each portion/week

Score: 9 or more Well done! You are meeting your fruit and vegetable and pulse target. This will help keep your heart healthy, and may help protect you from cancer.

Score: 0–8 You should include more fruit and vegetables and pulses in your diet. Aim for at least five portions of fruit and vegetables a day and four portions of pulses a week.

Carbohydrates	Score	
Breads	Wholemeal or rye bread	-1
	White bread/brown bread	-1
Breakfast cereals	Porridge, bran cereals, wholewheat cereals, sugar free muesli	+1
	Cornflakes, puffed rice, sugar coated or crunchy cereals, sweetened muesli and instant oat cereal	-1
Pasta/rice	Wholewheat/brown	+1
	White	-1
Bulgur wheat etc. couscous	One or more portions/week	+1
Cakes/biscuits	More than 2 portions/week	-1
Pastry/puddings	More than 2 portions/week	-1
Sweets/chocolates	More than 2 portions/week	-1

Score 0–4 Well done! You have a good intake of wholegrains and seem to limit your intake of refined starch products.

Score less than 0 You should reduce the amounts of refined starches in your diet and have more wholegrain products wherever possible.

Protein foods	Score	
Fatty red meat (beef, lamb, pork)	For each portion/week	-1
Lean red meat (beef, lamb, pork)	For each portion/week	0
Charred/well done meat (chicken, fish)	More than 2 portions/week	-1
Chicken/turkey	For each portion/week	0
Game i.e. venison	For each portion/week	0
Oily fish i.e. mackerel, salmon	For each portion/week	+2
White fish	For each portion/week	+1
Seafood, i.e. prawns, crab	For each portion/week	+1
Processed meat or meat products, i.e. salami, sausages, beef burgers,	More than 2 portions/week	-1
Eggs	0–6 eggs/week	0
	More than 6 eggs/week	-1
Omega-3 eggs,	For each egg/week	+1
Nuts	For each portion/week	+1
Soya products/TVP	For each portion/week	0

Score 0 or more Well done! You have a good balance of fish and meat in your diet, which gives you a good balance of unsaturated to saturated fats.
Score less than 0 You are having too much saturated animal fats and not enough omega-3 fats in your diet. You should aim to have equal amounts of fish as lean meat/poultry in your diet, try to include 2–4 portions of oily fish and 4 portions of pulses each week. Vegetarians may need to boost their omega-3 intake with flaxseed oil or supplements (see page 116).

Fats	*Score*	
Cooking oil	Olive/rapeseed (canola)/nut oil	+1
	Sunflower/corn oil	0
	Lard/butter	-1
Spread	Olive oil/soya spread	+1
	Sunflower margarine	0
	Butter	-1
	Low fat spread	0
Crisps/ savoury snack biscuits	More than 2 portions/week	-1
Shop bought biscuits/cakes	More than 2 portions/week	-1
Shop bought pastry/puddings	More than 2 portions/week	-1
Chocolate	More than 2 portions/week	-1

Score 0 or more Well done! You have a good balance of fats in your diet.
Score less than 0 You have a high intake of saturated animal fats in your diet.

Dairy products	*Score*	
Milk	No milk	-1
	Sheep/goats milk	-1
	Full fat milk	-1
	Semi-skimmed or skimmed milk	+1
Cheese	No cheese	-1
	0–4 oz (110 g)	+1
	More than 4 oz (110 g)/week	-1
Cottage cheese	For each portion score	+1
Low fat yoghurt/ fromage frais	No low fat yoghurt or fromage frais	-1
	For each portion score	+1

Greek style yoghurt/ full fat fromage frais	More than twice/week	-1
Cream	More than twice/week	-1
Ice cream	More than twice/week	-1

Score 0 or more Well done! You have a good intake of low fat dairy products.

Score 0 or less You either have too many high (saturated) fat dairy foods in your diet or not enough dairy. You should include more low fat dairy products daily. Aim to have 2/3 pint/400 ml of semi-skimmed or skimmed milk with an additional portion of low fat yoghurt or cheese each day.

Drinks	*Score*	
Drinks (non-alcoholic)	At least 2 litres/8 drinks/day	+1
Alcohol	More than 14 drinks/week	-1
Fizzy drinks	For each glass of regular (non-diet) drink	-1
	For each glass of diet drink	0
Fruit juice	More than 2 glasses/day	-1

Score 0 or more Well done! You meet the recommendations for fluids.
Score less than 0 You need to think about the drinks in your diet. Do you need to drink more fluids, cut back on alcohol, fizzy drinks or fruit juice?

Salt	*Score*	
Salt	If you add salt to food	-1
Ready meals or processed food?	More than twice a week	-1
Takeaway meals	More than twice a week	-1
Salty snacks	More than twice a week	-1

Score 0 Well done! You seem to be controlling the amount of salt in your diet.
Score less than 0 You currently eat too much salt. Cut back on ready meals, takeaways and processed food, and do not add salt to food.

The importance of exercise

BEING ACTIVE offers protection from breast cancer. Fifteen out of 20 high quality studies all agree that exercise is protective against breast cancer. These studies, which were recently reviewed in depth, show breast cancer risk is 30 to 40 per cent lower among women who take regular exercise.[64] This is comparable with the risk reduction seen with licensed breast cancer prevention drugs such as tamoxifen. Lack of exercise is thought to account for as much as 9 per cent of breast cancer cases and 14 per cent of bowel cancer cases in Western societies.

Exercise at any age seems to have a beneficial effect; best estimates suggest each additional hour of exercise a week during adolescence reduces later breast cancer risk on average by 3 per cent.[65] For pre and post-menopausal women beneficial effects are achieved with moderate or vigorous activities, such as brisk walking, swimming, jogging and cycling for three to four hours (30 to 45 minutes, five times) a week. Most studies show the best risk reduction by staying active throughout life, in other words during adolescence, adult years and after the menopause.

Being active clearly protects women from gaining weight, which is one of the biggest risk factors for breast cancer. The benefits of being active go beyond weight control. Exercise may protect women from breast cancer by influencing a number of key reproductive and hormonal factors linked to breast cancer risk; helping to delay menarche (onset of periods) until after the age of 12; and possibly increasing the likelihood of irregular menstrual cycles, thus reducing the total number of periods a woman experiences in her lifetime (see page 44).

Exercise also promotes a better hormone balance in the body. The Physical Activity and Total Health Study by Dr Anne McTiernan at the Fred Hutchinson Center, Seattle, USA tracked the effect of the recommended 45 minutes of exercise five times a week on levels of the cancer causing hormones oestrogen, testosterone and insulin in 170 women aged 55 to 75. After one year women who had been regularly exercising, lost small amounts of weight (3 pounds/1.4 kilograms), but also dropped their level of insulin by 17 per cent whether they lost weight or not. Exercise encourages cells to take up sugar from the blood-stream and lowers the need for insulin. Exercise also boosts the drop in oestrogen and testosterone seen with weight loss. Levels of hormones were 8 per cent lower in women who lost weight and also exercised, compared to those who simply lost weight.[66] Exercise also has fundamental effects on cancer growth and development, since it may be anti-inflammatory and stimulates the activity of the key gate keeper in cancer cells known as nuclear factor kappa b, which means cells are less likely to multiply, more likely to die and less likely to spread.

Exercise reduces the risk of breast cancer in women of all shapes and sizes, but has its greatest benefits in women of a healthy body weight, rather than in overweight women. The combined strategy of limiting calorie intake, increasing exercise and, above all, limiting weight and stores of body fat offers the greatest hope of protection from cancer.

Regular exercise also makes people feel better about themselves and is linked to a whole host of other health benefits. For example, regular exercise halves the risk of diabetes, and reduces risk of heart disease and stroke by 25 to 30 per cent. It is also one of the most important ways of keeping bones healthy, preserving the bone density and reducing the risk of developing osteoporosis in later life (see page 117).

There is no doubt that exercise is invaluable, but it is important to bear in mind that even if you exercise regularly, you cannot eat what you want and still lose fat. Successful fat loss relies on burning off 500 calories on a daily basis – that equates to 2 hours walking or 1½ hours of aerobics! Significant fat loss can only be achieved when you watch your diet – and exercise.

How much and what type of exercise?

There have been a series of confusing exercise recommendations over the past few years. Any increase in activity will be beneficial to your health and will help to control your weight, but the suggested targets for exercise are outlined below.

To maintain good health, prevent breast cancer and prevent weight gain you should take at least three to four hours of moderate exercise per week (for example, 30–45 minutes, five times per week). Moderate exercise includes brisk walking, swimming, jogging, cycling and dancing.

You should also include resistance training and flexibility exercises at least twice a week to help maintain your muscles. Muscles are the power house of the body and where many calories are burnt off. This will help preserve your metabolic rate (helping to prevent weight gain), improve your strength and stamina, and make you feel more conditioned. Resistance training and flexibility can be achieved with weight training or gym conditioning work.

These recommendations are ideal if you are currently trying to lose weight. If you have successfully lost weight it seems that trying to do at least an hour of moderate activity each day (seven hours per week) gives the best chance of keeping your weight down. Once you have got the exercise habit is it is important to keep it up. The health benefits are soon lost if you give it up; unhealthy rises in insulin are seen within three days of bed rest, and within ten days if a previously trained individual stops exercising!

Most people are not at risk of overtraining, but it is worth being aware that it is possible to do more exercise than is good for you. High intensity training in excess of two hours per day is not recommended, since this may compromise your immune system, and make you more prone to injury, inflammation and oxidative stress.

How to get moving

If you need motivation or are new to exercise you will find the following advice and exercise plans useful.

The first thing you need to do before getting active is to sit down and take a long hard look at your lifestyle. Write down what a normal day consists of over a period of one week and how and where you could incorporate 20–30 minutes of activity into your day – initially twice a week, building up over a period of 12 weeks to five sessions a week. For example, in weeks one to four build up from one to three sessions per week; in weeks five to eight try to do three to four sessions per week; in weeks nine to 14 do four sessions per week, with five sessions a week from week 14 onwards. During weeks 14 to 24 you should gradually increase the duration of activity to 45 minutes. Make an appointment with yourself to be active – put these sessions in your diary and check if you are keeping up with the programme at the end of each week. (See sample exercise plan on page 131.)

Your aim is to achieve the two types of fitness that are important for health: aerobic (which improves the health of our heart and lungs and helps us burn fat) and neuromuscular (which improves muscular strength, flexibility, muscular endurance and co-ordination skills). Remember, as well as providing strength, muscles burn off calories in the body, so retaining good muscle mass helps maintain a higher metabolic rate, and weight control.

Aerobic exercise

Many people chose to start with walking, as this is one of the most effective and cheap ways to get fit and burn fat off. Training with someone else is a very good motivator – recruit a friend or family member. Put you heart rate monitor on (see opposite) and aim to work within your fat burning zone (i.e. 60–65 per cent of your maximum heart rate) during the first few weeks. Other moderate aerobic intensity activities include cycling for pleasure, step machine, rowing, golf, swimming, mowing the lawn, etc. As you get a bit fitter you may want to build in some more intense aerobic activities such as running at 5 mph, hockey, squash, tennis, badminton, hard cycling, intense circuit training, hill walking and so on.

'We all underestimate the role of diet and lifestyle – I believe that these two factors are the key to good health. I have recently changed my diet because I found that my immune system was low, and improving my diet subtly has allowed me to get the optimum performance in my sport. We can all improve our diets with small changes that produce big results! I truly feel that living a life that consists of good food and exercise is what makes us strong. We don't have to follow an Olympic training regime but we should all make an effort to exercise a little each day. Whether it be taking the stairs instead of the elevator or walking a few hundred metres instead of taking the bus, life is too important for us not to embrace it.'

Jo Fenn
Olympic athlete

The benefits of using a heart monitor

It is a good idea to get into the habit of measuring your heart rate when you exercise. This is the best way to assess the safety and effectiveness of your exercise programme. Your heart rate is the number of heart beats per minute, which is an index of how hard your heart is working to pump blood through your body. You can measure your heart rate by simply feeling your pulse in your wrist or neck but it is better to use a heart rate monitor, as they are more accurate, and can give you a reading while you are exercising. Each monitor has a chest strap which is worn directly next to the skin as close to the heart as possible and a wrist watch-like receiver, which gives you a reading of your heart rate.

Exercising at different heart rate zones (intensities) has different health effects. Your maximum heart rate (MHR) is the fastest possible rate that your heart is capable of beating in one minute. You cannot, and should not try to exercise at this level. For fat burning and increasing the overall fitness of your heart and lungs it is best to work at 60–85 per cent of your maximum heart rate (this is your target heart rate). If you are just getting started you may find it easier to work at 50–60 per cent of your maximum heart rate for the first few weeks before building up the intensity. Building your

Heart rate zones at different ages

Age	Maximum heart rate (beats per minute)	Target heart rate i.e. 60–85% MHR
20	200	120–170
30	190	115–160
40	180	110–150
50	170	105–145
60	160	95–135
70	150	90–130

exercise programme on target heart rates is a built-in regulator for improving your fitness. As you do more training, especially if you lose weight, you will be able to perform the activities you did at the start at a much lower heart rate. This means you will need to do more work to achieve your target heart rate; that is you will gradually do more exercise as you get fitter and will keep building on your fitness.

In order to work out your target heart rate, you first need to work out your MHR using the following formula (as maximum heart rate decreases with age an age-related formula is used): MHR = 220 – your age. So at 30 years old your maximum heart rate would be 190 beats per minute (220–30 = 190).

Your target heart rate (THR) is 60–85 per cent of your estimated maximum heart rate: so for a 30-year-old woman with MHR of 190 her THR would be 115–160 beats per minute.

Exercise safely

Before beginning an exercise programme note the following:

• Consult your doctor if you have any medical conditions which may be affected by exercise, i.e. heart, circulation, chest or joint problems.
• If you are a breast cancer patient currently receiving or have received chemotherapy or radiotherapy within the past six months you should also consult your doctor before embarking on any exercise programme and follow the additional guidelines given on page 132.

- Build your exercise programme up slowly to reduce the likelihood of injuries.
- Always wear loose comfortable clothing and footwear with a good arch support.
- Don't eat a big meal before exercise; wait at least one hour after eating before exercising.
- Don't exercise if it is too hot or cold.
- Don't exercise if you are unwell.
- Drink plenty of water during and after exercise.
- Always warm the body up before exercising: gently run or march on the spot to raise your pulse, then mobilise all your joints (movements should start small, moving through the full range of motion) before stretching all the main muscle groups.
- Always stretch on finishing training.
- Don't over-exert yourself; signs of overexertion include nausea, sickness, dizziness, light headedness and chest pain.

Get-active plan for women wanting to reduce their cancer risk

	Week	Frequency (sessions per week)	Intensity (target heart rate – % MHR)	Duration (min)
Beginning	1	1–2	60–65%	15–20
	2	2	60–65%	15–20
	3	3	60–65%	20–25
	4	3	60–65%	25–30
	5–7	3–4	65–70%	25–30
Improvement	8–14	4	65–70%	30–35
	15–18	5	70–75%	35–40
	19–24	5	75–80%	35–40
Maintenance	24+	5	80–85%	40–45

Getting active for breast cancer patients

For the most part keeping active is safe and a recommended part of treatment and recovery. Start out gradually by including short spells (5–10 minutes) a few times a day. You should not exercise beyond 65 per cent of MHR during treatment, and limit your heart rate to 80 per cent of MHR or less in the six months following treatment.

Some women having chemotherapy can suffer short term drops in their blood cell counts. A drop in the level of platelets to below 50,000_/L (less than 1/3 of normal level) means you stand a much higher risk of bruising or bleeding and should only do gentle exercise and stretching.

You should also avoid exercise and consult your doctor if you have an irregular or high pulse (over 90 beats per minute), chest pain, dizziness, blurred vision, recent onset bone pain, paleness and anaemia, illness with fever, muscle weakness, sudden onset shortness of breath or unusual fatigue.

Women diagnosed with breast cancer tend to lose muscle mass due to the effects of treatment or inactivity. Rebuilding this muscle mass is an important step on the road to recovery, reducing fatigue, helping to preserve the metabolic rate and control weight. Patients

Get-active plan for women receiving treatment for breast cancer

Week	Frequency (sessions per week)	Intensity (target heart rate – % MHR)	Duration (min)
1	2	50–60%	5–10
2	2	50–60%	10–15
3	3	60–65%	10–15
4–7	4	60–65%	10–15
8–10	5	60–65%	15
11–12	5	60–65%	15–20

Get-active plan for women recovering from breast cancer treatment

Week	Frequency (sessions per week)	Intensity (target heart rate – % MHR)	Duration (min)
1	5	60–65%	15–20
2	5	60–65%	20
3	5	60–65%	20
4	5	60–65%	25
5–7	5	60–65%	25
8–10	5	65–70%	25
11–12	5	65–70%	30
13–15	5	70–75%	30
16–24	5	75–80%	30

who have had breast surgery and/or reconstruction, especially if it involves the lymph nodes in your armpit, should seek advice from their surgeon, physiotherapist or specialist nurse before embarking on a resistance exercise programme. You may find starting with a short set, for example one set of five repetitions, is a sensible starting point.

Resistance training

Once you are well on your way to getting fit (after 2 to 3 months) try to incorporate some resistance work each week (1 or 2 sessions of 30 minutes is all you need). If you are a member of a gym then use resistance training machines as opposed to free weights, as they provide both safety and novelty. Alternatively, buy a set of dumbbells and a simple book with illustrated exercises. When you first begin resistance training use light weights (about 1 kg/ 2 lb) and start with 3 sets of 15 repetitions with a breather in between – the goal is to fatigue your muscles within the last repetitions of the second and third set. Once you can achieve this, move onto heavier weights

'The beauty of physical exercise and a healthy eating plan is they become easier to follow the minute we decide to accept them as part of our lifestyles. My days of being at the peak of international sport are well and truly over, and since then, I, like many individuals have had to admit that it's not always easy to get off the sofa and exercise.

My biggest tip would be to accept and embrace exercise and a healthy eating plan as part of your lifestyle choice. In the four years since I retired from international athletics, I've remained motivated to keep in shape by varying my exercise plan, and have included boxercise, cycling, yoga, walking, skiing, rowing and of course running. The best way to keep on track is to keep your exercise challenging, make it exciting and allow yourself treats within your healthy eating plan.'

Diane Modahl
Commonwealth Games medal winner

with 3 sets of 8–12 repetitions. Challenge your body by increasing the workload as the exercises become easier.

Strength levels vary from one person to another so if you find the above weights too light then you may want to use the 'RM' technique to help you judge the most appropriate weight for you. One RM is the amount of weight an individual can lift with correct form for one repetition only; 8RM is the amount of weight that you can lift eight times only and so on. Make sure you breathe out as you contract your muscles i.e. the hard part of the exercise.

Following the correct order of muscle groups for resistance training is important. The larger groups (i.e. in the chest and back) should always be trained before the smaller muscle groups (i.e. the biceps and triceps in the arms). If smaller muscle groups were trained first, the larger groups could not then be trained to their full potential because smaller muscles would fatigue first (i.e. triceps should not be trained prior to bench pressing since they could limit the training effort for the main muscle group involved, i.e. pectorals). You may find the following sample trainining session useful if you have access to a gym (the staff should be happy to demonstrate the exercises).

Sample resistance training session for a complete beginner
(all exercises 1 set of 15RM):
Chest: bench press, pec deck
Back: lat pull down
Shoulder: shoulder/military press
Arms: bicep curls, triceps push downs
Legs: hamstring curl, leg extension, standing calf machine

Summary

- *Taking regular exercise reduces breast cancer risk by 30 to 40 per cent.*

- *Lack of exercise accounts for 9 per cent of breast cancer cases and 14 per cent of bowel cancer cases in Western societies.*

- *Three to four hours (30–45 minutes, five times a week) of moderate or vigorous activities such as brisk walking, swimming, jogging or cycling a week is recommended.*

- *The best breast cancer risk reduction is seen in women who are active throughout their lives; during adolescence, adult years and after the menopause.*

- *Exercise provides greater cancer protection in women of a healthy body weight, rather than in overweight women.*

- *Exercise protects against cancer through improving the hormone balance in the body and directly influences the function of cells, to make cancer cells less likely to develop and survive and spread.*

8

Sensible diet and lifestyle choices for breast cancer patients

IF YOU PRESENTLY HAVE or have already had breast cancer, you will wish to do all you can to keep well and to limit its chances of recurring. It has already been mentioned that better treatments and earlier detection mean many women respond well to treatment and remain cancer free. The odds of staying cancer free can be extremely high; for post-menopausal women detected early and receiving conventional treatment only 5 of every 100 women will relapse in five years. Odds are not quite as high for younger women who often present with more advanced disease, where 25 out of 100 will relapse within five years of being diagnosed. The previous pages outlined the steps women can take to prevent breast cancer occurring in the first place, which may have got you thinking about your own diagnosis and lifestyle. The most important thing is not to blame yourself for your diagnosis and dwell on factors that you are worried may have increased your risk in the past. Now is a good time to try to take control of your own destiny. An increasing body of evidence suggests that wise diet and exercise choices and weight control can markedly reduce your chance of a recurrence (particularly for younger women) and help guard against other conditions, such as heart disease, diabetes and osteoporosis. This section offers guidelines to cope with treatments for breast cancer and highlights lifestyle choices to stay well, and become fitter and healthier.

Types of cancer

Thirty per cent of women diagnosed with breast cancer from a mammogram have a cancer known as DCIS (ductal carcinoma in situ). DCIS is an early stage of cancer where cells inside the milk ducts of the breast have started to turn into cancer cells, but have not spread elsewhere outside of the ducts. The majority of women diagnosed with breast cancer have a more advanced stage known as invasive breast cancer where cancer cells break out of the ducts and move into the rest of the breast and can spread around the body. One out of every three women with DCIS will go on to develop invasive cancer if it is left untreated. Current practice is to remove the DCIS surgically; this may be followed by radiotherapy or hormone treatment. Professor Bundred and his team at the South Manchester University Hospital are currently researching the best treatment for DCIS.

Treatments for breast cancer

Most breast cancer patients have some form of breast surgery followed by a short course of radiotherapy, or six to eight months of chemotherapy or five years of hormone therapy, or a combination of these treatments. Seventy per cent of breast cancers are promoted by the hormone oestrogen and are known as oestrogen receptor positive (ER positive) tumours. Your medical team will have established if your tumour is one which is dependent on oestrogen, which tells them whether your tumour is one which can be successfully treated by drugs that block oestrogen. Chemotherapy is often used for tumours that are not oestrogen responsive, or in younger patients or where the cancer has already or is likely to have spread beyond the breast.

The most well-established hormone therapy is tamoxifen, which blocks oestrogen promoting cancer development and growth by preventing oestrogen from binding to the breast cells. More recent and potentially more effective hormone therapies are increasingly used in post-menopausal (but not premenopausal) women. These drugs reduce levels of oestrogen in the body by blocking the production of oestrogen from testosterone by aromatase in fat cells in the body. These aromatase inhibitors include anastrozole, exemestane and letrozole. Drugs that switch off periods are used in younger women. The commonest of these drugs, Goserelin (Zoladex), is a monthly injection.

The drug therapy Herceptin (trastuzumab) has received much publicity. This drug does not help all breast cancer patients but is specifically targeted for the 20 per cent of breast cancer patients whose cancer has large amounts of a particular receptor on the cell surface (the HER2 receptor), which transmits a signal from outside to the inside of the cell to promote cell growth. Most doctors will test your tumour to establish whether you have this receptor. Herceptin is currently licensed for women who have cancer that has spread beyond the breast. Recent studies have shown it may help women with early stage breast cancer when used alongside chemotherapy, with a staggering 46 per cent reduction in recurrence. This drug is not widely available at present in the UK but is under review.

Chemotherapy side-effects

If you are having chemotherapy it can knock your appetite for a few days, after which it quite quickly returns to normal. Some of the drugs actually boost your appetite, so if you find yourself eating more choose low fat and calorie food and drinks. Chemotherapy is designed to target fast dividing cancer cells in the body but may also cause short-term damage to other normal rapidly dividing cells, which line the mouth, gut and bowel (these are normally replaced every two days). This can cause a sore mouth, nausea, dry mouth, taste changes and constipation or diarrhoea.

Nausea is often well controlled with anti-nausea medication. The smell of cooking and food can sometimes make nausea worse. Many women find simple cold foods easier to manage. Popular choices include crackers, dry toast, yoghurt, rice pudding, cottage cheese, canned fruit and melon. Ginger and mint are well known for their anti-sickness powers; try mint tea, stem ginger or ginger ale. The feeling of an empty stomach can make nausea worse; eating small, frequent meals may be helpful.

Some women can experience changes in their sense of taste, which can make certain foods unappealing. Women tend to react differently, some preferring bland foods, while others will enjoy sharp tasting foods like pineapple or grapefruit. The best advice is to experiment with different foods and flavours. If you experience a metallic taste in your mouth, particularly with foods such as meat, you may find marinating meat with fruit juice helpful.

To help with a sore, dry mouth, keep your mouth clean and fresh using a soft toothbrush and mouthwash after you have eaten. Choose soft textured, mild flavoured foods and avoid acidic, spicy foods, and let hot foods cool before eating them. Foods you may find soothing include yoghurt, custard, ice-cream, frozen yoghurt, frozen canned fruit, banana, melon, papaya, cottage cheese and fruit smoothies, made with milk.

Some types of chemotherapy can cause diarrhoea. In the short term it may be helpful to cut back on wholegrain and fruit and vegetables. If drinking milk makes diarrhoea worse you may have become temporarily lactose intolerant. Use lactose reduced milk or over the counter lactose digestive aids (see page 96), which are widely available. You should try to include foods that help regenerate the healthy gut cells and bacteria in your bowel such as probiotic drinks and foods that contain soluble fibre. Banana, rice starch, oats and aloe vera may be helpful. Make sure you drink plenty of fluids. Conversely, pain killers or anti-sickness medications, or being less active, may make you prone to constipation. Constipation can often be resolved by drinking lots of fluids, increasing fibre in the diet from wholegrain foods, cereals, fruit and vegetables, and being active.

There is some evidence from animal studies that diets rich in omega-3 fats may improve the response rate of chemotherapy and radiotherapy. This is of course far from proven in human patients. In the mean time the high omega-3 Genesis diet is recommended (see page 167, for suggested intake).

Long-term effects of breast cancer treatment

Fatigue affects 70 to 100 per cent of women with breast cancer. It is a well-known side-effect of chemotherapy, radiotherapy and hormone therapy. Unfortunately it is not unusual for fatigue to persist long after treatments have finished; a third of patients complain of fatigue at least three years after treatment. It is important to reassure women just how common fatigue is and, most importantly, that it is rarely a sign that cancer therapy is not working or that the cancer is progressing. Some patients may be anaemic and may respond to treatments that boost their blood count. Patients are commonly advised to conserve their energy levels and to take extra rest and sleep. There is little evidence to support this advice and counter-intuitively the best chance of overcoming fatigue is to try to maintain or if possible increase amounts of activity and manage levels of stress (see page 52).

Weight control

Weight is certainly a major issue for many women diagnosed with breast cancer. You may be one of the six out of every ten women diagnosed with breast cancer who actually gain weight after being diagnosed. The reasons for weight gain among breast cancer sufferers are not entirely understood. Perhaps counter-intuitively weight gain is a particular problem for women receiving chemotherapy. My own research, published in the *Journal of Breast Cancer Research and Treatment* in 2004, suggested that higher intakes of calories, being less active due to fatigue and the lower metabolic rate associated with certain chemotherapy treatments were contributory factors.[67] Those women receiving hormone therapy may not see a difference in their weight on the scales, but may be conscious of putting on a few inches around their middles and a tightening of their waistbands, as they may experience a redistribution of fat stores. As well as being a concern to patients, doctors are also keen to try to help breast cancer patients manage their weight since there is strong evidence this may help reduce the chances of breast cancer reoccurring. A 2005 study by researchers at the Harvard Medical School found being 3 stone (19 kilograms) above your ideal weight may as much as double chances of recurrence,[68] while women who gained 1 stone (6.3 kilograms) or more in weight after diagnosis were one-and-a-half times as likely to relapse. These adverse effects of weight on relapse were seen in particular in women below the age of 50. Controlling weight may help reduce chances of relapse among older

Norma's story

Norma was diagnosed with breast cancer at the age of 46. She had a mastectomy and reconstructive surgery, and was prescribed a five-year course of tamoxifen. Three years later, she has learnt to cope with her illness by learning as much as she can about it and taking advantage of the moral support offered by patient groups.

At 5 foot (1.5 metres) and weighing 10 stone 3 lb (64 kg), Norma carries about 1 stone (6.4 kg) of extra body fat.

'When I was diagnosed no one at the hospital raised the issue of diet or watching your weight. Now that I am aware of their importance I think more carefully about my diet, which reassures me that I am doing everything in my power to keep myself well.

Since beginning the diet, I have managed to lose about a quarter of the fat that I need to shed. It hasn't been easy as I've found it difficult to control my weight since my diagnosis. I certainly wasn't as active in the early days and exercise is still not easy for me, as I am one of the few who suffer with muscle and nerve pain in my back following my reconstruction. I do try to go to a keep-fit class once a week, and go walking, but because I can't do a great deal I need to be more careful with my diet.

I did my fair share of comfort eating because of the breast cancer and my back problems, but I now think so much more about what I eat, avoiding all the high-fat takeaways, pasties and curries that I used to eat. I also think a lot more about how much I actually eat, so smaller plates that are piled higher with vegetables are gradually becoming a feature in our house. The great thing about the diet is it has made the whole family conscious of what we eat. I have a daughter who is 19, and I want to make sure she does all she can to avoid this disease.'

women too. A recent study, which generated plenty of interest, presented at the American Society of Oncology in 2005, showed that diet and weight control may help avert relapse from breast cancer. In this tightly controlled study 975 women following a low fat, fruit and vegetable-rich diet who controlled their weight during the first five years of diagnosis were 24 per cent less likely to relapse than women who ate a normal American diet and who gained the normal few pounds of weight. Weight control is crucial to limit the likelihood of other conditions arising, including other cancers, such as cancer of the womb, heart disease and strokes. A 2003 report from the National Surgical Adjuvant Breast and Bowel Project (NSABP) clearly showed how being 2 to 3 stone (12.7 to 19 kilograms) overweight meant breast cancer patients were 60 per cent more likely to develop other cancers including cancer of the womb as well as other diseases, and were 50 per cent more likely to succumb to these diseases in the four years after diagnosis.[69]

Weight control is particularly important for breast cancer patients. As well as hopefully reducing your chance of breast cancer recurring, weight control has other benefits for your future health. Not only will watching your weight make you feel better and more confident, but your chances of developing heart disease, diabetes and other cancers such as cancer of the womb will plummet.[70]

Hot flushes

If you are one of the many breast cancer patients who suffer with hot flushes you will not need reminding how debilitating and troublesome these can be. The sudden feeling of heat in the face, neck or chest is the classic symptom of the menopause, associated with lower oestrogen levels. Many breast cancer patients endure hot flushes; younger women who suddenly enter the menopause while undergoing chemotherapy, and older women who have worsening symptoms when they stop taking hormone replacement therapy (HRT) or when they use anti-oestrogen hormone drug treatments. The most effective treatment for hot flushes remains HRT, but many doctors are unwilling to prescribe HRT to breast cancer patients and the safety of alternative hormone therapy Tibolone for breast cancer patients is currently being assessed in the LIBERATE Study.

Many breast cancer patients choose to take natural remedies that have oestrogen-like effects, such as soya or isoflavone supplements like red clover, vitamin E and agnus-castus. Some women claim relief from hot flushes with these supplements, but they do not help the majority of women. There are also real concerns that they may reduce the effectiveness of hormone therapies such as tamoxifen and the newer hormone therapies, the aromatase inhibitors. Another herbal agent, black cohosh, is generally not advised; it is not a convincing agent for hot flushes, there are concerns it may enhance the toxic effects of some chemotherapy drugs and in animal models it accelerated the progression of cancer. There is also little data to support the use of natural remedies such as topical wild yam, evening primrose oil, ginseng or the Chinese herb dong quai. General healthy lifestyle tips such as weight control, regular exercise, relaxation, slow deep breathing and stopping smoking may help control symptoms and at worst they are good for your long-term health. Some women may find avoiding triggers such as hot temperatures, alcohol, hot drinks, caffeine and spicy foods helpful. Some interesting research by one of the scientists at Genesis, Professor Nigel Bundred, suggests some benefit from taking flaxseed; there was a 59 per cent reduction in hot flushes when women switched from taking a placebo to taking a flaxseed supplement.[71] Other medications your doctor may recommend include gabapentin and venflaxine paroxetine, which act on the nervous system and the brain, and may reduce flushes by 20 to 30 per cent.

Supplements and remedies

Many breast cancer patients are keen to use herbal remedies and nutritional supplements. There are absolutely no grounds for considering these over conventional treatment. Would you really consider passing up treatment that has been proven to work in favour of something that has no evidence to back it up? Many women opt to take natural remedies and supplements alongside their conventional treatment, thinking they will get the best of both worlds. You should think carefully about using natural remedies and you should certainly discuss these with your doctor. Many natural remedies are not as safe and effective as you may think. Many are ineffective, but a bigger concern is that some may also interact with your prescribed drugs and could actually do you more harm than good. Medications your doctor prescribes, such as chemotherapy and other drugs, work best within a narrow dose range; too much of these drugs may cause unpleasant or dangerous side-effects, while too little may not actually have the desired effect at all. Some natural remedies can affect the rate at which drugs are processed and removed from the body, which can either increase or decrease the levels of your prescribed drugs in your blood. Natural remedies such as garlic and ginseng, for example, reduce clearance of drugs and increase blood levels and toxicity, while ginkgo, echinacea and grapeseed increase clearance and may lead to under-dosing of drugs. St John's wort, which has known benefits for depression, may reduce the effective dose of chemotherapy by as much as half! The table on the following pages outlines some of the claims and concerns regarding natural remedies.

There is no evidence either that vitamin supplements help protect from cancer developing in the first place or from it recurring. High doses of vitamins, especially of the antioxidant vitamins C and E, and beta-carotene and selenium, are of particular interest among women receiving radiotherapy and some forms of chemotherapy. These treatments rely on producing free radicals to destroy cancer cells. Logically these supplements could be expected to help and minimise free radical damage to normal cells and reduce side-effects, and be of benefit. There is some worrying evidence from both human and animal studies that by mopping up these harmful free radicals, high levels of antioxidant supplements may limit their damage to the cancer cells and the effectiveness of these treatments. Thus taking antioxidants at the time of chemotherapy or radiotherapy may either boost or hinder its effects, and the outcome for any combination of antioxidant and therapy is hard to predict. Given that antioxidants may reduce the effectiveness of conventional treatment, it seems prudent to avoid using non-prescription antioxidants until more evidence becomes available. This does not mean you should limit your fruit and vegetable intake; it seems safe to eat up to ten servings per day. If your appetite is poor for more than a few days during treatment you may wish to take a general multivitamin and mineral supplement, which is fine provided it contains a standard amount of vitamins, or no more than 200 milligrams of vitamin C, 70µg of selenium and 15 milligrams of vitamin E.

Natural remedies for breast cancer patients, their health claims and concerns

Remedy	Health claim	Concern
Co-enzyme Q10	'Boosts immune system'	May reduce effects of radiotherapy
	Antioxidant	Interacts with warfarin to reduce blood clotting
Echinacea	'Boosts immune system'	Increased clearance of chemotherapy agents
Essiac	Anti-cancer	No harmful effects documented
	'Boosts immune system'	No evidence of anti-cancer effects
Omega-3 fish oils	Anti-inflammatory	Interacts with warfarin to reduce blood clotting
	May limit muscle wasting	
	Improves appetite	
Garlic	Anti-cancer	Interacts with warfarin, aspirin and other anti-inflammatory drugs to reduce blood clotting
		No evidence of anti-cancer effects
Ginkgo	'Boosts immune system'	May protect cancer cells from effects of chemotherapy
	Antioxidant	
Ginseng	'Boosts immune system'/tonic	Some oestrogen effects Interacts with some chemotherapy agents
		May affect blood pressure
Golden seal	Anti-cancer	Decreased metabolism of Paclitaxel chemotherapy may lead to toxicity
		No evidence of anti-cancer effects
Grapeseed	Antioxidant	May protect cancer cells from effects of chemotherapy
Isacador/ mistletoe	Anti-cancer	No evidence of anti-cancer effects
	'Boosts immune system'	

Remedy	Health claim	Concern
Kava	Promotes relaxation and eases menopausal symptoms	Toxic to liver
Amygdalin	Targets cancer cells	Cyanide toxicity
Milk thistle	Dyspepsia	Decreased metabolism of some chemotherapy may lead to toxicity
	Protects liver	Interaction with warfarin reduces blood clotting
	Anti-cancer	Can stimulate breast cancer growth!
Mushroom therapies	Anti-cancer	No evidence of anti-cancer effects
	'Boosts immune system'	Potential toxic effects
Selenium	Anti-cancer	Toxic if > 400 µg/day
	Antioxidant	
Shark cartilage	Prevents cancer spreading	No evidence of anti-cancer effects
		Not clear if the active proteins are absorbed in oral supplements
		Toxic side-effects in a recent study
Soya	Anti-oestrogen	May reduce effect of tamoxifen
St John's wort	Anti-depressant	Increases clearance of chemotherapy agents, may reduce effective dose by up to 50%

Exercise

Exercise may be difficult and unappealing, especially if you are someone who has never really enjoyed exercise. This is particularly true if you have had breast cancer and may be tired, anaemic, sore or weak after surgery; it is little wonder that most breast cancer patients become less active once they have been diagnosed.

Exercise has so many health and anti-cancer effects, and not surprisingly taking regular exercise after diagnosis seems to limit recurrence of breast cancer. A recent report from the Nurses' Health Study in the USA showed breast cancer patients who exercised for three or more hours a week (walking, jogging, cycling and callisthenics) were 30 to 40 per cent less likely to relapse from breast cancer in the eight years after diagnosis than women who were not as active. You will find specific guidance on exercise on page 132.

Bone health

It is important to think about the health of your bones since if you have had breast cancer, you may be more at risk of osteoporosis than you might imagine. Those at highest risk of osteoporosis include the many women who go through an early menopause during breast cancer treatment, or women taking one of the new generation of hormone treatments, the aromatase inhibitors, such as anastazole, exemestane and letrozole. Your doctor may monitor the thickness of your bones with a bone scan, or may ask you to take drugs to help boost their density. Sensible lifestyle choices to help preserve bone density are important for breast cancer patients, such as maintaining your intake of dairy products to boost calcium and vitamin D, doing regular weight bearing exercise and eating plenty of fruit and vegetables (see page 117 for more on healthy bones).

Lymphoedema

Lymphoedema is a chronic swelling that occurs in breast cancer patients when the normal fluid drainage channels of the lymphatic system are damaged during surgery or radiotherapy, so fluid (called lymph) collects in the arm and does not drain in the normal way. Lymphoedema occurs in about one in five women but is becoming less common because specialists now try to avoid giving women both surgery and radiotherapy to the armpit. Lymphoedema can start at any time after you have been treated for breast cancer, particularly if your arm becomes infected.

If lymphoedema does develop you will need treatment from a specialist nurse to push the excess fluid back out of your arm. This involves wearing a special elastic sleeve or bandage, and often having a special type of massage called manual lymphatic drainage. There is also some evidence that weight loss can help reduce symptoms. A recent study undertaken at the Royal Marsden Hospital, London by Dr Clare Shaw found swelling decreased significantly in women who were following a weight-reduction diet.

Summary

- *Between 70–100 per cent of breast cancer patients suffer with fatigue – staying active and managing stress reduces fatigue.*

- *Around 60 per cent of women gain weight after being diagnosed with breast cancer.*

- *Gaining a stone (6.3 kilograms) or more in weight may increase risk of relapse by as much as 50 per cent in women aged below 50.*

- *Weight control reduced risk of recurrence by 25 per cent in post-menopausal women.*

- *Breast cancer patients who are 2–3 stones (12.7–19 kilograms) overweight are 60 per cent more likely to develop other cancers, as well as other diseases such as heart disease.*

- *Engaging in moderate activity for three or more hours a week reduces risk of recurrence by 30–40 per cent.*

- *Many natural remedies are not safe and effective and may reduce effectiveness or increase the toxicity of your prescribed anti-cancer drugs.*

- *Breast cancer patients are often susceptible to osteoporosis and should follow recommended lifestyle advice (see opposite).*

- *Weight loss may help reduce the symptoms of lymphoedema.*

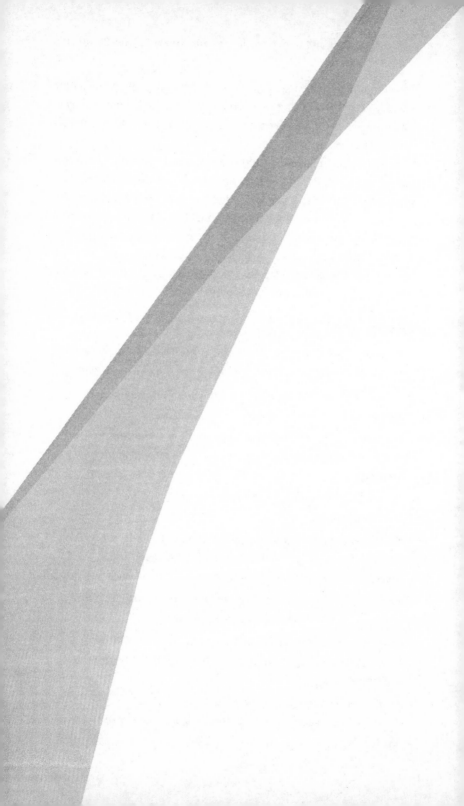

PART THREE

The Genesis Breast Cancer Prevention Diet

9
The overweight and obesity problem

THERE HAS BEEN AN EPIDEMIC of weight problems throughout the world over the past 25 years, and it is still out of control. The USA still has the dubious distinction of being one of the world's fattest nations, but many countries, including the UK, Australia, New Zealand and even parts of Africa, are fast catching up with the Americans. It is probably best to let the statistics speak for themselves. Rates of overweight and obesity have soared for both men and women. Back in 1980, 30 per cent of women in the UK were estimated to be overweight (BMI 25–29.9, at least 1½ stone/9.5 kilograms overweight) or obese (BMI 30 or over, at least 3 stone/19 kilograms overweight). Current estimates classify 60 per cent of all women in the UK as overweight; 22 per cent are obese. The average woman is now 1½ stone (9.5 kilograms) heavier than she was 20 years ago and officially about 1 stone (6.3 kilograms) overweight! A similar story has been played out in Australia where rates of overweight and obesity went up from 30 to 53 per cent; 21 per cent of women are now obese. If we continue to grow at this rate we can expect 80 per cent of all adults to be overweight or obese by 2035!

A worrying aspect is the massive increase in childhood obesity, which has reached epidemic levels in developed countries. Thirty per cent of girls under the age of ten in the UK are already overweight and 13 per cent are obese. In South Africa 25 per cent of girls are overweight by the age of 19.

Countries that seem relatively immune from the overweight epidemic are France, Italy, Holland and Belgium, where only 10 per cent of adults are obese. It is probably no coincidence that people in these countries are all passionate about food and cooking. They do not rely on ready meals or takeaways, which are loaded with fat. They opt for quality of food not quantity. Portions are on average about half the size of those in the UK.

The historic gap between men's and women's life expectancy is set to vanish in the UK. Males born in 2002 could expect to live to 76 while their sisters would live to 81, but by 2010 life expectancy of newborn males and females will converge at about 81. Experts believe the levelling of life expectancy between men and women reflects the large numbers of women who are overweight, and the increase in heavy drinking and smoking amongst young women. These factors make women prone to breast cancer as well as diseases traditionally experienced by men, such as heart disease.

Weight gain and the increased risk of disease

It has already been explained how weight gain increases your risk of breast cancer. It will not surprise you to read that weight gain also increases your risk of many other diseases, such as heart disease, stroke, diabetes and other cancers, including cancer of the womb and bowel. As you can see from the chart opposite, gaining just 1 stone (6.3 kilograms) in weight can significantly increase your risk of many diseases. Gaining more than 3 stone (19 kilograms) since the age of 20 means that you are three times as likely to have heart disease, five times more likely to have a stroke and 12 times more likely to develop diabetes!

As with breast cancer, not putting on weight is the best way of avoiding these diseases. For those who have already gained weight, do not despair! It is unlikely that you will return to the weight you were at the age of 20, but it is important to try and get nearer to this weight and at least to make sure that you do not gain any more weight. You have already seen that loss and maintenance of just ½ stone (3.2 kilograms) can reduce your risk of breast cancer by as much as 40 per cent, but it can also reduce your risk of diabetes by

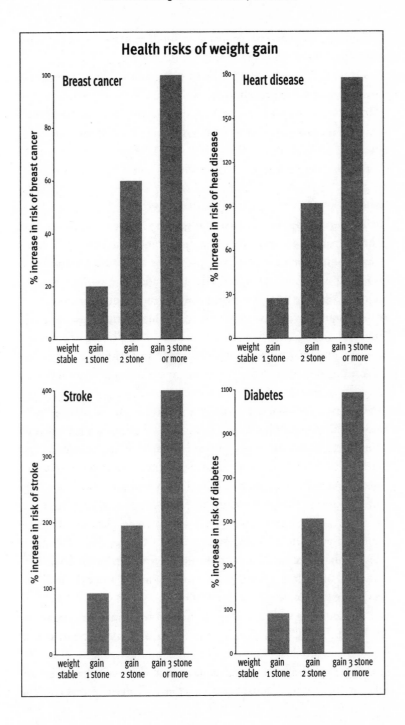

as much as 60 per cent, drop your blood pressure 5 per cent and cholesterol by 5 per cent.

Overweight is set to overtake smoking as the main preventable cause of illness and premature death in many Western nations. Being 2 to 3 stone (12.7 to 19 kilograms) overweight shortens life expectancy by seven years, which is the same amount as smoking: smoking and obesity together is seriously bad news and lowers life expectancy by 13 years.[1]

Energy in, energy out, energy stored

It has already been explained that gaining fat stores seems to be a normal part of getting older for many women. Energy comes from the consumption of foods. Excess fat is the body's energy store. Fat is laid down when a person is taking in more energy than they are burning off. The energy that is burnt off on the other hand is used to maintain the organs of the body (brain, heart, lungs, etc.) and the millions of chemical reactions that take place in the body; this is known as your metabolic rate. Some energy is used in the digestion of food and the rest is burnt off during any exercise or physical activity.

Contrary to what many people think, heavier people actually have a higher metabolic rate than thinner people. Many people think that eating too much fat leads directly to gains in body fat. In fact, taking in too many calories, whether they come from fat, alcohol, starchy or protein foods will be stored as body fat. To burn off excess body fat (your energy stores) you need to take in less energy than you are burning off. The only way to do this is to eat fewer calories, burn off more calories through exercise, or ideally both. One pound of stored fat contains about 3,500 calories. So to lose 1 pound of fat in a week you will need to have a 500 calorie deficit each day (500 kcal x 7 days = 3500 kcal).

The gains in weight and girth around the world are the result of higher calorie intakes and lower levels of activity. Higher energy (calorie) intakes are the major culprit, largely due to increased food portion sizes. This is particularly true of popular high fat, sugary or salty snack foods; many are twice or even three times the

Daily changes in diet or exercise	Change in fat stores over one year
Have an extra glass of wine	Gain 8 lb (3.6 kg)
Have an extra bag of crisps	Gain 17 lb (7.7 kg)
Have 2 extra biscuits	Gain 15 lb (6.8 kg)
Walk an extra 20 minutes	Lose 10 lb (4.5 kg)
Take the stairs instead of the lift (3–4 times/day)	Lose 6 lb (2.7 kg)

size, and providing two or three times as many calories as they did 30 years ago!

Most people could significantly improve their health by becoming more active. A quarter of the UK population is classified as sedentary (inactive), taking next to no exercise, with a further 50 per cent taking insufficient exercise to derive any real health benefit. This means that three-quarters of the population will not be burning off much energy, which will make it easier for them to gain weight. Being sedentary is actually a health risk in itself. A recent study found people who watched more than four hours of television a day were 25 per cent more likely to have high blood pressure than those who limited the number of hours on the sofa! If you recall, you should aim to take at least three to four hours of moderate exercise each week (i.e. 30–45 minutes, five times a week), such as brisk walking, swimming, jogging, cycling and dancing. Once you have successfully lost weight, you should probably try to fit in an hour a day (i.e. seven hours per week) of moderate activity to stand the best chance of keeping that weight off. So, instead of settling down in front of the TV to watch a film, why not get out for a walk to help you to relax, feel better and burn off 600 extra calories at the same time.

Weight gain can be the result of gradual changes in the balance between energy intake and energy you burn off and it can take place over many years. The table above shows the changes in fat stores over the course of one year that can go along with small changes to your diet or levels of exercise.

Liz's story

Liz is a 33-year-old mother with 2 young children. She was unfit, overweight (at 14 stone 10lb/92.7 kg and with a BMI of 32) and suffered from headaches linked to a weight-related condition known as benign intercranial hypertension. Liz started on the diet plan 2 years ago and has managed to lose 27 pounds/12 kg in weight and drop 4–6 dress sizes. She now weighs 12 stone 11 lb/80.5 kg (BMI 27), is clothes size 14 and has a waist measurement of 29 inches/72 cm (healthy range).

'Most of my weight was lost in the first six months, but it is still slowly coming down. If I had not decided to change my ways two years ago, who knows, I probably would now have been more like 18 stone than nearly 2 stone lighter. Like many women, my weight problems began after getting married and settling down. I was a very active child and teenager; a competitive swimmer. Since settling down and having children my weight has been on the up. Thanks to the diet and my regular exercise routine I now feel so much happier and confident in myself and have so much more energy. I even weigh a little less than I did when I got married, and most importantly now have the energy and self-confidence to take the kids swimming again.

I have found the diet easy to follow; it is very clear and you know exactly what you should be having, the type of food and the amounts. I love my regular exercise – I go to mini-trampolining classes. The first week was hard as I stuck rigidly to the diet but only managed to lose a pound. But sticking with the diet and exercise really paid off over the following weeks. You start to feel and look healthier over the first month and you really do feel so much better that it is easy to believe you are so much more in control of your future health, and doing all you can to protect yourself from cancer. I just feel so much better in myself. This has got to be the greatest motivation to stick with it.'

Risky times for weight gain

There are times when putting on weight seems particularly likely. Forewarned is forearmed. Watch out for these and try not to lose control of your weight:

- Marriage or settling down with a partner is a classic time when women may start to overeat. They often find themselves eating as much as their partners despite often having much lower energy requirements.
- Pregnancy is an obvious time of weight gain for women, many of whom find it difficult to return to their pre-pregnancy weights, particularly with the erratic meal patterns and lack of time to exercise that often accompanies motherhood.
- Giving up smoking makes people put on weight, typically ½–1 stone (3.2–6.3 kilograms). Stopping smoking is the best thing smokers can do for their health and well-being (see page 48).
- Stress and emotional upsets can have very different effects on appetite and weight. Some people overeat at times of stress and put on weight, while others lose their appetite and lose weight.
- Studying or long working hours often lead to weight gain. This is not surprising as these spells involve many hours sitting still at the computer, with erratic meal patterns and often high intakes of calorie-rich snack foods.
- The calendar has its fair share of regular favourites for weight gain with Easter, summer holidays and, of course, Christmas festivities, which often seem to extend over a number of months. On average, people eat an extra 175,000 calories over Christmas and gain 5 pounds (2.2 kilograms) in weight, with accompanying rises in blood pressure and cholesterol levels.
- A number of drugs increase the tendency to put on weight, such as steroids, many anti-depressants, oral contraceptives, beta-blockers and some anti-convulsants. Many women believe hormone replacement therapy causes weight gain, but there is little evidence to suggest that HRT leads to any weight increase in addition to that normally gained at menopause.

Is your weight a health risk?

Simply weighing yourself on a set of scales will not tell you if you are a healthy weight. You need to take three factors into account to decide whether you need to try and lose some weight: (1) the amount of weight you have gained since the age of 20; (2) your body fat level; and (3) your waist measurement. If you have experienced any increase in these factors, then weight loss may be your key to better health.

Note down these three factors now, as they apply to you:

(1) How much weight have you gained since the age of 20?

(2) What is your body fat level? Remember: you can assess your body fat using a bioelectrical impedance meter or the Genesis Body Fat Ready Reckoner, which estimates your body fat from your weight and hip measurements (see page 72).

Weight reduction drugs

Given the vast numbers of overweight people across the world, it is no surprise that pharmaceutical companies are attempting to develop drugs to help people lose weight. Two drugs, Orlistat (Xenical Roche) and Sibutramine (Reductil, Abbott), can currently be prescribed in the UK in well-defined circumstances, usually only if an individual is at least 2 stone (12.7 kilograms) over-weight and has an existing medical condition that requires them to lose weight. Neither of these drugs is a magic bullet, and like most drugs they may have side-effects. These drugs do not take the place of energy restricted and exercise weight loss plans, but simply help to boost their success. Orlistat limits absorption of fat (calories) in the bowel, while Sibutramine helps control the appetite and maintains metabolic rate during dieting. Newer drugs that act simultaneously on the appetite, gut and fat cells are currently undergoing evaluation.

(3) What is your waist measurement? Remember: your waist is a good proxy of your stores of harmful abdominal fat. Measure your waist at the level of your belly button with a tape measure, while standing and breathing out.

How do you measure up?

	Adult weight gain	Percentage body fat	Waist
My measurements			
Healthy range	No more than 10 lb (4.5 kg) in weight should be gained during adult life	20–28%	32 in (80 cm) or less

Summary

- Sixty per cent of all women in the UK are overweight; 22 per cent are obese.

- The average woman in the UK is now 1½ stone (9.5 kilograms) heavier than she was 20 years ago and 1 stone (6.3 kilograms) overweight!

- To lose 1 pound (0.45 kilograms) of fat in a week you will need to eat 500 calories less each day than you are burning off.

- Higher energy (calorie) intakes are the major culprit for the rise in weight, largely due to increased food portion sizes.

- Twenty-five per cent of the population do no exercise at all and 75 per cent will not burn off enough energy to control their weight.

- Risk times when women often gain weight include settling down, pregnancy, studying, hectic work lives or times of stress.

10
The Genesis weight loss and weight maintenance plans

Weight loss or weight maintenance?

IF YOU HAVE ALREADY GAINED TOO MUCH WEIGHT, have a higher than desirable body fat level or waist measurement, or indeed all three, the advice and suggested diet plans beginning on page 167 will help you lose weight.

If you are a healthy weight it is crucial you stay that way. To maintain a healthy weight you will still need to watch your diet and keep up at least seven hours of moderate exercise per week. A weight maintenance plan can be found for you to follow on page 176. Both the weight loss and weight maintenance plans are healthy, balanced, calorie-controlled diets, which are rich in cancer protective foods. To choose the correct plan, simply chose the appropriate plan for your body weight. The planner tells you the calorie intake and the number of servings of starchy, protein, fruit, vegetables, dairy and fat foods and occasional treats allowed within the plan. Use the list on page 169 as a guide to the amounts of food allowed in each serving. Before looking at the specifics of the diet it's important to examine some of the issues you need to consider before beginning the diet.

Weight loss

Losing weight at any point in your life can make you feel better about yourself and can dramatically improve your health. It has already been stated that experts agree losing just ½ stone (3.2 kilograms) and keeping this weight off means you reduce your risk of developing diseases, such as breast cancer, diabetes and heart disease, and can improve your state of mind. It has already been mentioned how women who managed to lose 5 per cent of body weight in the recent Genesis weight loss survey experienced significant improvements in hormone levels. Those women who managed to lose 5 per cent of body weight also experienced significant improvements in mental (14 per cent) and physical (11 per cent) well-being scores.

The Genesis weight loss plan requires you to make permanent changes to the way you eat and to take more exercise. Sometimes there are factors in life that make it difficult to make significant changes and hamper efforts to lose weight. Before launching into the programme, think about whether it is a good time for you to try and make these changes. The key elements to think about are as follows:

- Do you have support from friends and family?
- Will any friends/colleagues/family join the programme with you to offer moral support?
- Do you have a lot of stress in your life at the moment?
- How confident are you that you will be able to make changes to your diet?
- How confident are you that you will be able to fit regular exercise into your daily life? Think about the time, the opportunity you have and your motivation to do more exercise.
- What weight loss are you hoping to achieve? Will you be happy to lose 1 to 2 pounds (0.45 to 0.9 kilograms) of fat a week?
- Make a list of the positives of trying to lose weight at this time. How will weight loss make you feel better?
- Try to think of the negatives of trying to lose weight at this time. Can you think of any ways in which losing weight may be a problem to you?

After thinking about these factors, you may decide this is not a good time to lose weight. If you are not sure you are sufficiently motivated to lose weight you may wish to remind yourself of the health benefits of weight loss (see page 63). If you are under stress, can you do anything to help manage this? Can you get more support? Can you find time to exercise? If you still don't think this is the right time, consider making the changes at a later date when the time is right for you.

If you think you are ready, you now need to think about how you see yourself and your body image and set yourself some realistic goals.

Body image

Your body image is how you view your size, shape and appearance and how you feel about them. Few people are totally happy with their appearance, especially those with a weight problem; indeed most people have a list of things they would like to improve. For some, negative feelings about their appearance knocks their confidence and self-esteem so much it affects the way they live their lives. Doctors working in weight control know all too well that these negative feelings must be overcome before any attempt at dieting can be made. Feeling negative makes it extremely difficult to implement healthy lifestyle changes and lose weight. You may find it helpful to stop and think about how you see yourself, especially if you are someone who is preoccupied and worried about your appearance. Take some time to think about the issues below. This will be time well spent, as it can only improve your chances of diet success.

- It is worth being realistic about the weight you are likely to achieve when you follow the diet. You may have to accept that you are unlikely to be as slim as the fashion image you aspire to be. Accepting a realistic healthy weight for yourself means you are much more likely to succeed.
- Try to think more positively about yourself: list four things you like about yourself as a person; list four things you like about your appearance; try to think of four overweight people you like or respect – what do you like about them?
- Try to think differently: if you have ever been particularly upset about your size think about what happened and how you ended up feeling; try to think about how you could have handled the situation better.
- Think of four things you would like to do but have been putting off because of your weight or lack of confidence.

- Try to think of things that would make you feel better about yourself, apart from losing weight.
- Look after yourself. Giving yourself a reward is a great way to start feeling better about yourself. You need to get used to the idea that you are worth pampering and spoiling. Why not take some time for you? Have a long bath, take time out to read a book, listen to music or watch a film, book a massage or facial, go for a walk, do yoga, go dancing, gardening, have a new haircut or go shopping with a friend.

Margaret's story

Margaret is in her late 40s and is a busy GP and the mother of four children. There is a strong history of cancer in her family: both her mother and grandmother died from breast cancer; her mother at the age of 60 when Margaret was in her early 30s. Three of her uncles have also had prostate cancer, suggesting a likely genetic fault in the family, although this has not been identified. Margaret's weight had crept up with each pregnancy and the pressures of looking after her family, which left her little time to fit in regular exercise or be vigilant over her own diet. Margaret weighed 10 stone 10 lb (12.7 kg) and her BMI was 24. However, she had gained nearly 2 stone in weight since she was 18 years of age. Margaret lost 10 pounds (4.4 kg) of this body fat over 12 months of following the diet and exercise plan, losing 2½ inches (6 cm) from her waist and halving her level of testosterone.

'Obviously as a doctor I am conscious of the importance of a healthy lifestyle for promoting and maintaining good health. As a busy mother and full-time worker I am more than aware that any lifestyle choices must fit in to everyday family life. Women of my age find themselves pulled by their roles in looking after the younger and older generations, leaving us little time to look after our own health. I managed to slot an extra walk into my daily routine. I still ate the same foods as the family but in smaller amounts. It is well worth weighing and recording the foods you eat for a short spell, to become aware of your normal patterns.'

Setting goals

Having established that you want to lose some excess weight (body fat) you need to set yourself some sensible targets. You need to be realistic about what you can achieve. A sensible target to start off with would be to aim to reduce your hip and waist measurements by 5 per cent and to reduce your body fat by 10 per cent. For example, if you currently weigh 12 stone (76 kilograms), have a waist measuring 38 inches (96 centimetres), hips measuring 44 inches (112 centimetres) and estimated fat mass of 62 pounds (28 kilograms), sensible targets would be to aim to lose 2 inches (5 centimetres) off both your waist and hips, and about 7 pounds (3 kilograms) of body fat.

Realistically, you will only lose 1 to 2 pounds (0.45 to 0.9 kilograms) of body fat a week with the plan. Fat loss can sometimes seem frustratingly slow but this is the best way to lose fat and keep it off. More rapid weight loss occurs at the start of any diet due to loss of water, which is bound up to energy stores in the liver and muscle, and not loss of body fat. Some lean tissue is always lost when weight is reduced. The Genesis weight loss plan is designed to help limit this inevitable loss, by being relatively high in protein and reminding you keep on exercising.

The Genesis weight loss plan

The Genesis weight loss plan is a healthy, balanced, calorie-controlled diet and exercise programme designed specifically for women who wish to lose body fat to reduce their risk of cancer (and other diseases). The diet is rich in cancer protective foods such as wholegrains, fish, low fat dairy foods, vegetables and fruit. It avoids foods high in saturated fat, which may increase cancer risk, to boost the cancer protective effects of weight loss. The plan is not intended for use by children and is not specifically aimed at men. The general recommendations of the healthy balanced diet and exercise that are promoted, but not the specific plan itself, will however be beneficial for the whole family. Women who are breast-feeding, pregnant or trying to become pregnant are generally not recommended to try to lose weight and thus should seek advice from a qualified medical practitioner. Likewise, if you are following a therapeutic diet, have a medical problem or take medication you should also seek advice from your medical practitioner before embarking on any diet and exercise programme, since losing weight may affect the required dose of some drugs.

No diet will work unless you keep to it. The weight loss plan can easily fit into your life and is relatively easy to follow, which is the proven key to success. The essential ingredients of the weight loss plan are to eat the right types of food, not eat too much and to take regular exercise. Remember that it is sensible to fill up on low calorie foods when you are trying to control your weight, but eating too much of any food, however healthy it is, will bring in too many calories and promote gains in fat. A recent study by Dr Che and researchers at the Barbara Ann Karmanos Cancer Institute in Detroit asked women at high risk of breast cancer to eat more fruit and vegetables. This actually resulted in them gaining about 5 pounds (around 2 kilograms) in weight! Having chosen the appropriate plan for your weight try and stick to the amounts of food recommended.

Weight loss plan

Daily portions	Current weight						
	< 9 st/ 57 kg	9–10 st/ 57–64 kg	10–13 st/ 64–82 kg	13–14 st/ 82–88 kg	14–16 st/ 88–101 kg	16–18 st/ 109 kg	> 18 st/ 113 kg
Calories	1300	1400	1500	1600	1700	1800	1800
kJ	5434	5852	6270	6688	7106	7524	7524
Carbs/ starch	6	7	7	8	8	9	9
Protein	6	7	7	8	9	10	10
Fruit	2	2	3	3	3	3	3
Vegetable	5	5	5	5	5	5	5
Dairy	3	3	3	3	3	3	3
Fat	3	3	3	4	4	5	5
Minimum litres fluid	2	2	2	2	2	2	2
Weekly extras	2	2	2	2	2	2	2

Food group and serving sizes

Starchy foods	1 serving
Wholegrain breakfast cereal	3 tablespoons, or 1 whole-wheat 'biscuit' cereal
Porridge oats, muesli	2 tablespoons
Wholemeal, rye bread	Medium slice or ½ roll
Wholemeal pitta bread/chapatti	½ large
Rye crispbread	3
Wholewheat cracker	3
Oatcake	1
Couscous/bulgur wheat,	30 g/1 oz uncooked 2 tablespoons cooked
Pasta/noodles/rice (preferably wholewheat or brown)	30 g/1 oz uncooked or 3 tablespoons cooked
Baked/boiled potato (in skin)	1 medium (115 g/4 oz)
Cassava, yam, sweet potato	1 medium (115 g/4 oz)
Wholemeal pizza base	Quarter of a thin medium pizza base
Sweetcorn	1 corn on the cob

Protein foods	1 serving
White fish	45 g/1 ½ oz
Canned fish in brine/tomato sauce	45 g/1 ½ oz
Seafood, prawns, mussels, crab	45 g/1 ½ oz
Oily fish, i.e. mackerel, sardines, salmon, trout	30 g/1 oz
Chicken, turkey	30 g/1 oz (i.e. 1 slice the size of a playing card)
Lean beef, pork, lamb	30 g/1 oz
Eggs	1 egg
Baked beans	2 tablespoons (60 g/2 oz)
Lentils or other cooked pulses	2 tablespoons (60 g/2 oz)
Quorn/tofu	60 g/2 oz
Textured vegetable protein	15 g uncooked
Low fat hummus	1 tablespoon

Vegetables	1 serving
Any boiled/steamed vegetables (except potato)	2–3 tablespoons
Salad	1 bowl
Homemade vegetable soup	1 bowl
Beans and corn	2 tablespoons
Vegetable juice	200 ml/7 fl oz

Fruit	1 serving
Oranges, pear, apple	1 fruit
Banana	1 small
Small fruits: clementines, apricots	2 fruits
Melon, pineapple	1 slice
Grapes, cherries	15
Berries	cupful
Dried fruit	3 dried apricots/ handful of raisins etc.
Fruit juice (unsweetened)	Small glass (125 ml/4 fl oz)
Stewed fruit (unsweetened)	3 tablespoons
Canned fruit (in natural juice)	3 tablespoons

Milk and dairy foods	1 serving
Milk (semi-skimmed or skimmed)	200 ml/7 fl oz
Yoghurt plain or flavoured low fat/ whole	1 small pot (150 g/5½ oz)
Fromage Frais (low fat)	2 tablespoons
Cottage cheese	½ pot (115 g/4 oz)
Cream cheese (low fat)	1 tablespoon
Cheese, preferably: reduced fat Cheddar, Edam, feta, Camembert, mozzarella	Matchbox size (30 g/1 oz)

Fat	
Olive or soya margarine	1 teaspoon
Olive or other monosaturated oil	1 dessertspoon
Oil-based dressing	1 tablespoon
Nuts and seeds	1 tablespoon
Avocado	¼ average pear
Pesto	1 dessertspoon

Occasional/extra foods*	1 serving
Crisps (low fat)	1 small packet (25–30g)
Nuts	½ small packet
Biscuits, plain	1
Chocolate	½ small bar or 1 fun-size bar
Beer or lager	300 ml/½ pint
Wine	125 ml/4 fl oz glass
Spirit and diet mixer	2 pub measures
Ice cream	1 scoop
Muesli/cereal bar	1
Malt loaf	1 slice
Scone	½ scone

*You may want to include other snacks or treat foods (see page 179)

Note: Dairy foods are an important part of weight loss and weight maintenance plans. If for some reason you are unable to have dairy products in your diet, you should replace them with 3 additional servings of protein foods and ensure that you take a daily calcium and vitamin D supplement.

The vital ingredients of the weight loss plan

This is a weight loss, cancer prevention plan. The key elements are:
- limits calorie intake and promotes weight loss
- promotes moderate or vigorous exercise for three to four hours per week (i.e. 35–45 minutes, five times a week)
- high in whole grains and low in refined carbohydrate
- high in omega-3 anti-inflammatory and monounsaturated fats, low intake of saturated (animal) and polyunsaturated fat
- low in alcohol
- rich in cancer protective fruit and vegetables and low fat dairy products
- relatively high in protein and fibre to boost feelings of satiety, and your ability to stick to the diet.

The elements of the weight loss plan will now be examined in turn.

Protein

Protein forms an essential part of any diet, as it provides the building blocks for muscles and organs in the body. Protein foods include meat, poultry, fish, pulses, nuts, soya and dairy products.

These foods are particularly important for someone trying to lose weight as they are filling and may help prevent some of the inevitable loss of muscle when people lose weight. A recent report studied varying amounts of protein in the diet and found that diets with the highest protein content (providing 30 per cent of energy) increased satiety, spontaneously reduced calorie intake by 400 calories a day and led to the loss of 11 pounds (5 kilograms) of body fat over three months.[2]

Make sure you include a protein food at each meal. Many of the protein foods recommended in the plan have a low fat content to limit calorie intake, such as fish, seafood, poultry and lean meat. Lean red meat can be included up to four times a week; it is one of the major sources of iron. Take care with grilled or fried meat, which may contain cancer causing chemicals. It is best to stew or braise meat wherever possible, or steam fish. You should also remember to trim meat of any excess fat before cooking and if using mince, dry fry it and drain off excess fat. Nuts and oily fish are higher in fat (and therefore calories) but are a vital source of the beneficial omega-3 fatty acids and should be included. Pulses are a great low fat, high fibre source of protein, which are also packed full of health giving nutrients. Soya foods can also be included, since the best available evidence suggests a neutral effect on breast cancer risk.

Dairy products

Many people leave out dairy products when they are trying to slim. Some dairy products, such as cheese, cream and butter, are indeed high in fat and calories, and should be avoided. Emerging evidence now suggests that low fat dairy products, such as semi-skimmed milk, cottage cheese and yoghurt are an important part of any diet; not only are they are low fat, high protein foods, but the high calcium content also helps control weight. Recent research from the Royal Veterinary and Agricultural University in Denmark showed a short term boost in calcium intake (1800 milligrams per day) cut the amount of fat absorbed in the gut by 70 calories a day. This would be enough to help you to lose 2.2 pounds (1 kilogram) of body fat over three months.[3]

Fruit and vegetables

Fruit and vegetables are an important part of any weight loss plan, especially vegetables, which are low in calories and a great way to fill up. Eating a large salad starter can stop you overeating; a recent study found dieters who ate a large salad before a pasta meal ate 12 per cent fewer calories for the overall meal. Fruit and vegetables are also packed full of vitamins and chemicals, which are vital for good health. For example, 4 pounds (1.8 kilograms) of broccoli has the same amount of calories as a small bar of chocolate, but the broccoli provides enough vitamin C for 20 days!

Fresh, frozen and salad vegetables should all be included in your diet. Limit salads containing mayonnaise, though you can use specified amounts of olive oil dressings. Avocados are a good source of healthy monounsaturated fats but are high in fat and calories and should be eaten in the moderate amounts as specified in the plan. Try to include fresh fruit each day; you can also have small amounts of fruit juice and dried fruit, but bear in mind these are higher in natural sugars and calories than fresh fruit.

Fat

Fat is loaded with calories and is a key issue for the slimmer. We have already seen that very low fat, high carbohydrate diets are not the answer (see page 84), but neither are the very low carbohydrate, high fat regimes that have been popular recently. Though great for short-term weight loss, these diets are often high in saturated fat and likely to have long-term consequences with regard to the risk of heart disease, osteoporosis, kidney stones – or indeed cancer risk. The Genesis diet does not take any of these approaches and is a moderate fat diet that is rich in monounsaturated and omega-3 fats.

Fibre

You have already seen how wholegrain foods are better for your health than refined foods. Including whole grains in the diet is also a great way of controlling calorie intake and weight. A 2003 report from Dr Liu and colleagues at the Nurses' Health Study looked at wholegrain intake in 74,091 American female nurses, aged 38 to

63 years. Their diet and weight change was tracked over 12 years between 1984 and 1996. Women who consumed more than three portions of whole grains a day were only half as likely to suffer major weight gain as women who did not include these in their diet. Women who consumed the most whole grains gained an average of 1.52 kg less over the 12 years than women with the lowest intakes.[4]

Processed and 'diet' food

Processed food and ready meals should not form part of your diet, as they are too high in salt and fats; particularly the unhealthy saturated and hydrogenated fats (see page 83).

Diet products are everywhere. Sometimes it seems that the fewer calories there are in a food, the more you are expected to pay for it! It is not recommended that you base your diet on foods that are marketed as 'diet' foods. Look at the box opposite for explanations of some of the labels you might find on diet foods. It is useful to be aware of the calorie content of foods. Read the calorie content of foods from the label. Don't forget that calories will usually be listed per 100 grams or per 100 millilitres of the product; you will need to multiply this up (or down) to tell you how many calories are in each serving.

Don't be fooled into thinking that all low fat foods are low calorie. A lot of low fat foods still contain large amounts of fat and therefore calories. A low fat claim simply means the food has less fat than the normal high fat version. Other low fat foods can be full of sugars and can provide just as many calories!

Supplements

There are plenty of supplements that claim to boost weight loss, for example chitosan and kelp. The benefits of such supplements are far from proven and are not part of this diet plan. Following this weight loss plan should ensure that you get the right balance of nutrients in your diet and do not need to take additional supplements. Some supplementation may, however, be needed if you are restricting your diet in some other way. Many women, especially those who eat little or no meat are deficient in iron, while women who have

Diet foods – read the label

Claim	Meaning
Low fat	No more than 3 g of fat per 100 g or 100 ml of product
Fat free	No more than 0.15 g of fat per 100 g or 100 ml
Low sugar	No more than 5 g per 100 g or 100 ml
Low calorie	Product has no more than 40 calories in a serving
Reduced calorie	Has 25% fewer calories than the standard product
Light/Lite/Diet	Does not mean anything
Reduced sugar	Has 25% less sugar than the normal product
No added sugar	No sugars added to the food
Sugar free	No more than 0.2 g per 100 g or 100 ml
High fibre	At least 6 g per 100 g or at least 6 g in a reasonable expected daily intake

low intakes of dairy products due to allergy or preference may require a calcium supplement. Taking large doses of single vitamins is not a good idea and may lead to an imbalance in other nutrients in the body and be hazardous for the health (see page 106).

Drinks

It is essential to try and drink plenty of fluids when you are trying to lose fat, particularly as you will be exercising as well. Many people do not drink enough. It is quite common to mistake thirst for hunger, which leads to overeating. Try to drink at least 2 litres (3½ pints) of fluid per day. Drink water, herbal tea and tea and coffee without sugar. Fizzy drinks are full of sugar (a glass of standard fizzy drink contains about 6 teaspoons of sugar) and calories but contain no beneficial nutrients. Occasional diet drinks may be incorporated into the diet plan. Alcohol is bad for breast cancer risk and is also fattening – a 250 ml glass of wine contains 220 calories (920 kJ)! Alcohol should be limited if you are trying to control or lose weight.

Weight maintenance plans

Use this table once you have reached your desired weight. It indicates the calories and food servings appropriate to your weight. The recommended foods and serving sizes are given in the Food Group Servings list on page 169.

This plan is designed to meet your energy requirements at your body weight, assuming you are achieving the recommended amount of activity. So it is crucial that you keep up the exercise. You should recheck your weight, body fat and waist measurement monthly; particularly during high risk of weight gain times (see page 159).

Here are some tips for keeping off the fat:

• keep monitoring your weight, waist and hips every four weeks
• follow the recommended plan to guide you towards the best types and correct amounts of food
• make sure you manage your stress levels
• keep up the regular exercise
• be aware of what and how much you are eating; be aware that portion sizes tend to drift upwards!

Daily portions	Current weight				
	‹ 9 st/ 57 kg	9–10 st/ 57–64 kg	10–13 st/ 64–82 kg	13–14 st/ 82–88 kg	›14 st/ 88 kg
Calories	1800	1900	2000	2100	2100
kJ	7524	7942	8360	8778	8778
Carbohydrate/ starch	8	9	10	10	10
Protein	10	10	11	12	12
Fruit	3	3	3	3	3
Vegetables	5	5	5	5	5
Dairy	3	3	3	3	3
Fat	5	5	6	7	7
Minimum Fluid litres	2	2	2	2	2
Weekly extras (max)	5	5	5	5	5

Successful weight loss and maintenance

The crux of any diet is to make sure that you do not overeat. The timing of meals can play a large part in how easy you find it to limit your intake. The optimum pattern will vary between individuals, but is most likely to be around three to four meals per day. It seems that people who try to divide their food into lots of smaller snack meals throughout the day inevitably eat more than they would when they have fewer larger meals. A recent study from the University of Nottingham in England showed that women eating their food over nine small meals ate 250 calories more than the same food split over three meals.[5] Having regular meals is probably a good idea for most people. Skipping meals may mean you are more likely to resort to high calorie snack foods later when you are really hungry. For some people, skipping meals in the day means they eat more calories in the evening than they might have done if they had eaten regularly throughout the day. Having breakfast may also be good for weight control. When healthy women were deliberately asked to miss breakfast they ate 100 extra calories throughout the day, and had a slight increase in cholesterol levels.[6] The size and frequency of meals does not appear to affect the way the body processes food. A number of carefully monitored studies reviewed by Professor Andrew Prentice from the MRC Dunn Clinical Nutrition Centre in Cambridge, England, concluded that the frequency of eating makes no difference to the efficiency with which fat is stored provided individuals eat the same number of calories in the day.

Some people think that food eaten late at night is more fattening, but it is not more likely to be stored as fat than food eaten earlier in the day. It is the total calories that are eaten in 24 hours that determines whether we lose or gain fat. A detailed study from the MRC Dunn Clinical Nutrition Centre confirmed a large evening meal was processed identically to the same food taken as several small meals throughout the day. A survey of 7000 American adults in the National Health and Nutrition Examination Survey (NHANES I, 1971–75) showed the proportion of energy consumed in the evening (after 5 p.m.) was not a significant predictor of weight gain over the next ten years.

Planning

Planning your meals and shopping will put you in control of your diet. Make sure you always have a supply of suitable healthy snacks (see opposite).

Gaining control over eating

For many people overeating has become a habit that seems difficult to break. You may be one of the many people who find that as soon as you start to follow a diet, you immediately want to eat more. Here are some tips to try and get your eating under control:

- Try to eat regularly.
- Don't skip meals and let yourself get too hungry. This may mean you ultimately overeat and consume more in that one later meal than you would have done in the missed and subsequent meal.
- Avoid the triggers that make you overeat, i.e. sweet foods such as chocolate, biscuits and cakes, or the sight and smell of favourite foods.
- Avoid the situations that make you overeat, i.e. watching television, boredom, being with certain friends or family members.
- Only eat when you are hungry, not just because you think it is a mealtime or because you are bored.
- Try and overcome the urge to eat and snack when you are not hungry. Distract yourself by engaging in another activity, e.g. go for a walk, phone a friend, have a bath. You should find that the urge to overeat will eventually disappear. The more times you resist the urge to overeat the weaker these urges should become!
- Drink plenty. You may think you are hungry when in fact you are thirsty, which can lead to overeating. Drinking water (particularly carbonated water) before a meal will fill you up.
- It takes 15 minutes for you to realise you are full when you have eaten. Try to wait at least 15 minutes after finishing a meal to decide whether you are actually still hungry and if you need seconds.

- Have plenty of vegetables and salad with the meal or start with a bowl of salad or vegetable soup to fill you up.
- Finish a meal with a hot drink, i.e. tea or coffee.
- Brush your teeth after a meal to stop the craving for sweet foods.
- A lot of people find it difficult to see food left on a plate. Don't be tempted to eat up any food left by other members of your family.
- Regular exercise is a good way of regulating your appetite.
- Try to have enough sleep. Overeating is more likely when you are tired and have erratic sleeping patterns.
- Sometimes you can be persuaded to eat by others. Be assertive and say when you do not want to eat or drink something.
- Don't eat or drink while doing something else. Don't eat while

Healthy snack foods

Most commonly available snacks are high in calories, fat and sugar and have no place in your weight loss plan. Here are some healthy, low calorie snacks you could try:
- grilled mushrooms on a slice of wholemeal toast
- baked beans on one slice of wholemeal toast
- vegetable soup
- vegetable juice
- salad or cooked vegetables with cottage cheese, low fat cream cheese or hummus
- piece of fresh fruit
- ½ pot of cottage cheese
- crispbread and cottage cheese or low fat cream cheese or hummus
- bowl of canned bean salad
- pot of yoghurt
- 30 grams (1 ounce) of nuts
- 30 grams (1 ounce) of dried fruit
- slice of malt loaf
- smoothie made with semi-skimmed milk and 1 piece fruit
- ½ can of sardines or pilchards

watching the television, standing up or catching up on emails, which can lead to overeating because you are not conscious of how much you are eating.

• Take time to enjoy your meals. Good food shouldn't be rushed.

Sample meal plans

If you would like some guidance on getting started on the diet, the following sample meal plans should help. You can follow them rigidly (though you may need to adapt the portions to suit your designated calorie intake – as these plans are for women following the 1300 calorie planner) or use them as a guide, swapping your favourite foods for those in the meal plans (as long as they are from the same food group and quantity). For example you can swap a 30 g (1 oz) cereal portion for 1 slice of wholemeal toast for breakfast. The meal plan for week 4 is for vegetarians but there is no reason why this cannot be followed by meat eaters too – you might enjoy the change!

The best pattern of meals will vary between individuals, but I recommend having 3 to 4 meals per day. You should try to include protein or dairy foods in all meals. Take a few minutes to think how your dinner plate normally looks. Many people have a plate that features lots of meat (model A, opposite) or lots of starchy food (model B). To fall in line with the recommendations of this diet, your meals should look like the plate in model C or model D. Half of your meal should be fruit or vegetables and the remaining half should be protein and starchy food, or it can be just protein for some meals. You can eat your meals whenever you wish. The plans also include a snack, which you can have at any time in the day that suits you. You'll notice that some of the snacks are quite substantial – this is perfectly acceptable as long as you stay within your daily calorie limit.

Here are a few key rules to remember when planning your diet:
• Aim to include equal amounts of fish as lean meat in your diet.
• Try to eat 2 to 4 portions of oily fish and 4 portions of pulses each week. Vegetarians may need to boost their omega-3 intake with flaxseed oil or supplements (see page 116).

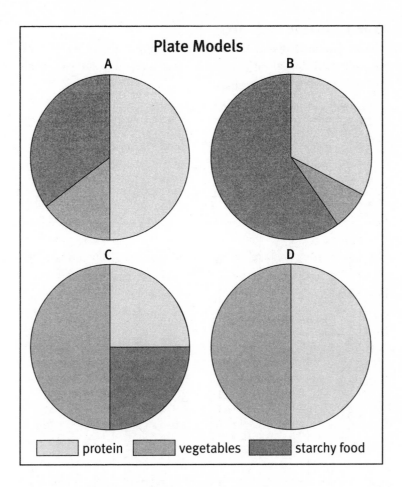

Plate Models

A   B

C   D

protein   vegetables   starchy food

- If you are still hungry on the plan you may have more vegetables, but try not to go overboard with fruit.
- Avoid having more than 6 eggs per week.
- Do not have more than 115 g (4 oz) of cheese per week.
- If you are unable to have dairy products in your diet, you should replace them with 3 additional servings of protein foods and ensure that you take a daily calcium and vitamin D supplement.

The four-week meal plan

Note: The meal plan is for women weighing less than 9 stone following the 1300 calorie planner. You can adapt it to suit your goals using the diet planner on page 168.

* indicates a recipe that is featured in this book

Week 1	Breakfast	Lunch	Dinner	Snack when required
Monday	Fresh Bircher Muesli* served with grated apple	White Bean and Barley Salad with Garlic and Yoghurt Sauce* green salad	Chicken Poached in Vinegar* 200 g (7 oz) mashed potato 3 portions vegetables Ginger Oranges*	1 piece of fruit
Tuesday	2 slices wholemeal toast with olive oil spread 2 grilled rashers lean bacon grilled mushrooms	200 g (7 oz) jacket potato 115 g (4oz) cottage cheese side salad 1 piece of fruit	Sesame-crusted Salmon with Asian Greens and Ginger Salsa* 6 tbsp brown rice 1 portion steamed vegetables	low fat yoghurt 1 piece of fruit
Wednesday	125 ml (4 fl oz) orange juice porridge made with 3 tbsp oatmeal and 200 ml (7 fl oz) milk	Lentil and Mushroom Soup* wholemeal roll and 1 tbsp low fat cream cheese 1 piece of fruit	turkey stir fry (115 g/4 oz turkey, 2 portions vegetables) 60 g (2 oz) boiled noodles	1 tbsp nuts and seeds
Thursday	Granola* served with 3 tablespoons low fat yoghurt and a cup of berries	2-egg omelette with tomatoes and 30 g (1 oz) Edam mixed salad 200 g (7 oz) potato salad with yoghurt dressing	Monkfish Plaki* large salad 60 g (2 oz) boiled brown rice	Broad Beans with Sauteed Tofu* 3 crispbreads
Friday	2 pieces of fruit and 2 tbsp fromage frais	tuna and corn pasta salad (115 g /4 oz can tuna mixed with 60 g /2 oz pasta, corn, peppers and 1½ tbsp yogurt) mixed salad vegetables	Roast Pepper Parcels with Spinach, Hazelnuts and Cottage Cheese* large salad 60 g (2oz) bulgur wheat	2 tbsp low fat hummus with raw celery, carrot, pepper (capsicum) 3 crispbreads
Saturday	Couscous with Apricots and Mango*	Griddled Sardines with Tomato Avocado and Lime Salsa* tomato salad pitta bread	Pan-fried Fish with Beetroot steamed green vegetables Balsamic Roasted Pears	1 tbsp nuts and seeds
Sunday	1 scrambled egg with 30 g (1 oz) smoked salmon 1 wholemeal roll	Root Vegetable Soup* cheese on wholemeal toast 1 low fat yoghurt or 2 tbsp fromage frais	115 g (4 oz) roast chicken salad 200 g (7 oz) roast sweet potatoes Apricot, Almond and Apple Salad*	Sicilian Salad of Fennel and Oranges* 1 oatcake

Week 2	Breakfast	Lunch	Dinner	Snack when required
Monday	Granola* served with 3 tbsp low fat yoghurt and a cup of berries	Marinated Mackerel with Cucumber and Dill Salad* wholemeal roll	115 g (4 oz) tandoori chicken (chicken coated in natural yoghurt mixed with tandoori paste then grilled) 60 g (2 oz) boiled brown rice 1 tbsp low fat yoghurt to drizzle mixed salad	1 tbsp low fat cheese 3 wholegrain crackers
Tuesday	½ grapefruit 3 tbsp sugar free muesli 200 ml (7 fl oz) semi-skimmed milk	Couscous Salad with Grapes and Pistachio Nuts* 60 g (2 oz) cooked chicken 1 low fat yoghurt	Tuna and Avocado Burgers* 1 corn on the cob, boiled tomato salad 1 piece of fruit	½ portion of Granola*
Wednesday	125 ml (4 fl oz) orange juice porridge made with 3 tbsp oatmeal and 200 ml (7 fl oz) milk	115 g (4 oz) cooked peeled prawns green salad 150 g (5½ oz) new potatoes 1 piece of fruit	Oyster Mushrooms in Ginger Sauce with Colcannon* steamed vegetables low fat fromage frais	½ can sardines or pilchards 1 oatcake
Thursday	grilled tomatoes 1 wholegrain bagel olive oil spread	jacket potato and baked beans salad 1 piece of fruit	oven-baked salmon Griddled Broccoli, Fennel and Radicchio* 60 g (2 oz) bulgur wheat	fruit smoothie made with 200 ml (7 fl oz) semi-skimmed milk and 1 piece of fruit
Friday	2 Weetabix 1 tbsp raisins 200 ml (7 fl oz) semi-skimmed milk	Cabbage, Turkey and Bacon Soup* wholemeal roll	Cottage Pie with Cauliflower Topping* 2 portions steamed vegetables Lemon and Watermelon Granita*	Bulgur Wheat, Chickpea and Grape Salad*
Saturday	Fresh Bircher Muesli* served with grated apple	Sweet Potato and Cream Cheese Pancakes* mixed salad	Steamed Halibut in Pak Choi steamed green vegetables 200 g (7 oz) boiled potatoes 50 g (1¾ oz) puy lentils fresh fruit salad	1 can vegetable juice
Sunday	Fromage Frais Pancakes with Honey and Blueberries*	Root Vegetable Soup* wholemeal roll with 90 g (3 oz) canned salmon 1 low fat yoghurt	Chicken with Grapes and Apricots* 60 g (2 oz) boiled brown rice mixed salad Mango Sorbet*	1 tbsp nuts and seeds

* indicates a recipe that is featured in this book

Week 3	Breakfast	Lunch	Dinner	Snack when required
Monday	1 piece of fresh fruit 30 g (1 oz) smoked salmon 1 tbsp low fat cream cheese wholegrain bagel	60 g (2 oz) cooked turkey with avocado, mustard and salad on 2 slices wholemeal bread spread with 2 tsp fromage frais	Roasted Fillet of Lemon Sole on Watercress and Sweet Potato Cake* steamed green vegetables	125 g (4½ oz) cottage cheese 3 crispbreads 1 tbsp nuts
Tuesday	½ mango fromage frais	Tuna with Beans* potato salad in yoghurt dressing tomato salad 1 piece of fruit	Chicken- and Tabbouleh- stuffed Pitta* Griddled Vegetable Salad*	30 g (1 oz) Granola* cereal with milk
Wednesday	Fresh Bircher Muesli* served with grated pear	Warm King Prawn and Endive Salad with Grapefruit and Peanuts* 150 g (5½ oz) new potatoes 1 low fat yoghurt	Pasta with Fresh Tomato Sauce* mixed with small can tuna 30g (1 oz) low-fat cheese, grated mixed salad	2 tbsp low fat hummus mixed raw vegetables
Thursday	Granola* served with 220 ml (7½ fl oz) milk 1 small banana	jacket potato with cooked chicken (115 g/4oz) in yoghurt dressing 1 tbsp nuts and seeds	Pumpkin, Chickpea and Coriander Curry* 60 g (2 oz) brown rice tomato salad 1 tbsp yoghurt Tofu with Ginger and Lime*	Asparagus and Avocado Soup* 3 crispbreads
Friday	porridge made with 3 tbsp oatmeal 200 ml (7 fl oz) milk cup of mixed berries	Spanish omelette with mixed beans (2 eggs and 2 tbsp beans) tomato salad	Pearl Barley Risotto with Crab and Chilli* mixed salad 1 piece of fruit	2 slices of malt loaf with a little olive oil spread
Saturday	Granola* with ½ grapefruit and orange with 2 tbsp low fat yoghurt	125 g (4½ oz) canned sardines on 2 slices wholemeal toast tomato salad	115 g (4 oz) roast chicken Carrot Gratin* steamed vegetables 200 g (7 oz) jacket potato Mango Sorbet*	125 g (4½ oz) cottage cheese mixed raw vegetables
Sunday	1 piece of fruit 2-egg omelette with 1 tbsp cream cheese and generous sprinkling of fresh herbs	Root Vegetable Soup* 2 slices wholemeal bread with olive oil spread 1 piece of fruit	Braised Fillet of Lamb* Roasted Root Vegetables and Broccoli* 1 portion steamed vegetables Rhubarb and Elderflower Jelly*	1 low fat yoghurt

* indicates a recipe that is featured in this book

Vegetarian	Breakfast	Lunch	Dinner	Snack when required
Monday	2 Weetabix 200 ml (7 fl oz) milk 1 small banana	White Bean and Barley Salad with Garlic and Yoghurt Sauce* green salad piece of fruit	Pumpkin, Chickpea and Coriander Curry* brown rice 3 tbs low fat yoghurt tomato and cucumber salad	200 g (7 oz) bean salad (beans and dressing)
Tuesday	1/2 grapefruit 2 slices wholemeal toast with olive oil spread baked beans (4 tbsp)	green pepper and cottage cheese omelette (2 eggs, 115 g/4 oz cottage cheese) tomato salad rice salad (30 g/1 oz rice)	Stuffed Courgettes with Pine Nuts and Wild Rice* crisp green salad 1 low fat yoghurt	low fat hummus with crudités
Wednesday	1 portion of Granola* 1 portion mixed berries 220ml (7½ fl oz) milk	Asparagus and Avocado Soup* wholemeal roll filled with 1 egg and watercress	Quorn bolognese (150 g/5oz) with tomato sauce 60 g (2 oz) spaghetti mixed salad Tofu with Ginger and Lime*	1 slice malt loaf with olive oil spread
Thursday	125 ml (4 fl oz) orange juice porridge made with 3 tbsp oatmeal and 200 ml (7 fl oz)milk	200 g (7 oz) jacket potato baked beans green salad	Napoleon of Aubergines, Celeriac and Goats Cheese* Bulgur, Chickpeas and Grape Salad* mixed salad	1 low fat yoghurt
Friday	Fresh Bircher Muesli* with 1 grated apple	Lentil and Mushroom Soup* wholemeal roll and low fat hummus	Tofu and Spinach Lasagne* butter beans low fat fromage frais	1 piece fruit
Saturday	2 slices toast scrambled eggs grilled mushrooms and tomatoes	Sweet Potato and Cream Cheese Pancakes* mixed salad	lentil chilli (115 g/4oz lentils 300 g/10z kidney beans wholemeal pitta mixed salad	Root Vegetable Soup* or can vegetable juice
Sunday	Mixed Berry Brushetta*	lentil chilli with jacket potato	Roast Pepper Parcels Couscous Salad with Grapes and Pistachios* mixed salad Ginger Oranges*	Broad Beans with Sautéed Tofu* 3 crispbreads

* indicates a recipe that is featured in this book

Common problems with following a weight loss plan

In the following pages you will find hints on how to deal with common problems encountered by dieters.

Breaking the diet

Successful dieters are a highly valued commodity! Scientists have made many attempts to distil the essence of their success. The most widely studied group are 4000 successful dieters on the National Weight Control Registry in the USA, who have lost at least 2 stone (12.7 kilograms) and kept it off for at least a year. They found that keeping on track during weekdays, weekends and holidays is a better approach than dieting more strictly on weekdays than at weekends and holidays, and such people are one-and-a-half times more likely to keep weight off.[7]

Everybody breaks their diet from time to time. Successful dieters in a recent study from the Weight Control and Diabetes Research Center USA reported eating foods that should have been restricted between three and five times a week. The most important thing to do if you slip up on your diet is to get back on track as soon as you can. A common response is to think you have undone all the good you have done and give up on the diet. If you do suffer a setback with your diet, don't give up. One in ten of the successful dieters on the National Weight Control Registry in the USA reported overcoming a small relapse where they had regained a few pounds, while those with larger relapses found it more difficult to get back.

Allowing yourself a prescribed diet break may be a good way to deal with high risk periods such as holidays or to combat boredom with the diet. An interesting study by Professor Rena Wing looked at the impact of a planned two-week diet holiday on diet success. After the break dieters managed successfully to return to their diets and it did not hamper their long-term success.[8]

Comfort eating

Many people overeat when stressed or depressed. Comfort eating is often little comfort in fact, particularly if you are trying to lose weight, and often leads you to feel more anxious and fed up. Try to manage stress in other ways through regular exercise, relaxation or complementary therapies, such as massage, reflexology, aromatherapy and yoga (see page 52).

Premenstrual syndrome

The week before the start of a period is a difficult time for many dieters. They often feel fed up, anxious and experience cravings for sweet and salty foods. The cravings are thought to be due to the body trying to take in enough carbohydrate to balance levels of chemicals in the brain. Try to meet these carbohydrate cravings with whole grains rather than refined carbohydrates. Magnesium is thought to help suppress these cravings; good dietary sources of magnesium are wholegrain cereals and vegetables. Fortunately, many women find they actually experience fewer premenstrual symptoms when they lose fat and take regular exercise.

There is also some evidence that calcium and vitamin D may prevent premenstrual syndrome. A recent analysis by Dr Bertone-Johnson among 1000 women within the Nurses' Health Study showed women with the highest intakes of calcium (> 1200 milligrams of calcium/day) and vitamin D (700 IU/18 µg) were 30 to 40 per cent less likely to suffer than women with the lowest intakes of these nutrients (500 milligrams/day calcium; 200 IU/10 µg vitamin D).[9]

Do you get SAD in winter?

Many people get a touch of the winter blues when they feel low and lethargic and are more likely to comfort eat. Some people are particularly susceptible and have what is known as seasonal affective disorder or SAD. There are an estimated half a million SAD sufferers in the UK. SAD is more common among women, particularly those aged between 20 and 50. Most of us fortunately don't get these extreme symptoms; however the winter blues and SAD are both caused by lack of daylight, which disturbs the chemical balance of the brain, reducing amounts of a substance called serotonin, which promotes relaxation and happiness. Starchy and sugary foods boost levels of serotonin. A craving for comfort foods, especially sweet foods, is the body's attempt to increase serotonin levels during the winter months. So what is the answer? Exercise is great therapy for SAD; it helps restore the chemical balance of the brain. Walking outdoors for one hour a day is a good prescription for SAD sufferers. Overcoming the inertia to exercise during winter, particularly outdoors, could make you feel a lot better about yourself, help curb those carbohydrate cravings and keep you on track on your diet plan.

Sleep deprivation and fatigue

Too much sleep and not enough exercise will not help your weight loss efforts, since sleeping is the time when the least calories are burnt off. You may be surprised to learn that lack of sleep may well be a contributory factor to weight problems. Lack of sleep is an endemic problem in modern society; many people want to eat when tired, in an attempt to recoup missing energy. Being short of sleep has been shown to disturb the hormone balance in the body, increasing levels of the appetite stimulating hormone gherelin and reducing levels of the hormone leptin, which tells you when you are full. Little wonder then, that being tired boosts the drive for food, which may make you overeat and gain weight. To sum up, you should make sure you get enough, but not too much sleep!

Food cravings

Many food cravings are linked to certain times or situations and have actually been learnt. Many people crave something sweet at the end of each meal as they were brought up with desserts or sweets. It is possible to try to reprogramme your brain to try to lose these urges. Some people find the urge will go away if they can distract themselves for 15 to 20 minutes. You might phone a friend, go for a walk, have a bath and clean your teeth. The more often you ignore these cravings, the more likely these are to fade away – good luck!

Slow or no fat loss while following the plan

If you feel you are not losing the predicted 1 to 2 pounds (0.45 to 0.9 kilograms) per week, check the following:

- Are you following the correct diet plan for someone of your weight (see page 168)?

Louise's story

Breast cancer was in Louise's family tree on both parents' sides, affecting two of her mother's cousins and her father's sister. Her own sister has also had breast cancer but has now been successfully in remission for six years. Louise's father died of lung cancer and her mother died of a rare form of skin cancer when Louise was just 18; this was when Louise started to comfort eat and to put on weight. Over the next 20 years Louise gained 8 stone (50 kg) in weight.

'There were many short-term attempts to lose weight over this time, you name it I had tried it. Whilst I always lost something on these diets it didn't stay off for long and now I realise they didn't tackle the root cause of my overeating. Finally, about four years ago, I joined the breast cancer weight loss research programme, which made me think about what may happen in the future if I didn't tackle my weight problem. At 15 stone 6 lb (97 kg) and 5ft 4 inches (1.62 m) I was classed as morbidly obese according to the BMI chart. I was lucky that my weight hadn't caused me any problems so far and felt ready to do something serious about it. The secret of successful dieting for me was to look at what I ate but also why I ate. I finally realised I had started to overeat for comfort when my mother died, and went on doing this through my life. Whenever things were not right I would turn to food. Now I look for another way to avoid the overeating cycle, like going to the gym, reading a book or having a relaxing bath. I no longer need food to comfort me. Recognising this was the key to sustained weight loss. I now feel in complete control; life seems more fun and I am so much happier with myself, its not just about how you look it is how you feel. I have reduced clothes size, my bust size has reduced 10 inches (25 cm), my waist 12 inches (30 cm) and my hips 10 inches. I have less fear of breast cancer. I now know I have done everything in my power to avoid it; if it happens now then I can't blame myself and can concentrate on beating it. Now that I have got to the weight I want to be I now have to concentrate on remaining here.'

- Are you actually following the recommended diet?
- Are you taking the recommended amount of exercise, i.e. three to four hours of moderate activity per week (30–45 minutes, five times a week), and resistance training and flexibility exercises at least twice a week? Don't miss out on any other opportunities to exercise in the day, take the stairs, walk to the shops, etc.
- Keep a food and activity diary for four days as a check to see what you are eating and to see how active you really are (see page 265). Try and include weekdays and weekends in your diary.

Keeping the fat off

The hardest thing about losing fat is keeping it off. Many successful dieters will have been here before, but will have managed to bounce straight back to their old weight once they stopped dieting. Many dieters know only too well the frustration of yo-yo dieting; keeping the fat off is the most crucial stage of dieting. If you go back to your old eating patterns and levels of activity, as it is so easy to do, you will simply and quickly have an excess energy intake. This excess energy will rapidly be stored as fat and you will quickly put all of the lost weight back on (see page 177).

To keep at your lower weight you will still need to watch your diet and keep up at least three to four hours of exercise per week (i.e. 30–45 minutes, five times a week), ideally increasing this to an hour a day to give you the best chance of keeping the weight off. You will find weight maintenance plans on page 176. These maintenance plans are still healthy balanced diets, but allow you slightly bigger servings of starchy and protein foods compared to your previous fat loss plans. To choose the correct fat loss maintenance plan, simply select the appropriate plan for your newly acquired lower body weight. The planner tells you the calorie intake and the number of servings of starchy, protein, fruit, vegetables, dairy, fat foods and occasional treats that are allowed. Use the food exchange list on page 169 as a guide to the amounts of food allowed in each serving. The plan is designed to meet your energy requirements at your new lower body weight, assuming you are achieving the recommended three to four hours of activity each week. It is therefore crucial that you keep up the exercise.

Check your progress

An important part of any weight loss plan is to monitor your progress, to check you are losing fat. It is recommended that, while you are following the diet plan, you weigh yourself and measure your waist and hip measurements once a week. You can record these in your monitoring sheet (see page 263). Use these weight and hip measurements to reassess your body fat levels every two weeks. If you are following the maintenance plan do this monthly.

PART FOUR

The Recipes

11
The recipes

WITH THE EXCEPTION OF A FEW of my own favourites, the recipes in this section have been selected and developed by Roy Ackerman and Silvena Rowe, two fabulous chefs who kindly volunteered their services. As you will soon discover the recipes are healthy, easy to prepare – and amazingly delicious.

Many people wrongly assume that losing weight and weight maintenance is all about denial – these recipes prove it is anything but! Good food that tastes great needn't be fattening – it is simply a matter of learning to use naturally delicious foods to their best advantage, utilising ingredients cleverly to maximise flavour, and, of course, keeping an eye on portion sizes.

As well as the standard nutritional information, each recipe tells you how many diet plan portions of protein, vegetable, fat or starchy carbohydrate it contains. This will make it easy for you to incorporate the recipes into the diet plan.

Some of the recipes have been developed with families in mind – these are tasty, exciting meals that adults and kids will love. These recipes are indicated by the letters Fm. Many people have more time to spend on their meals at weekends, and recipes which are suited to those days or if you have guests, are indicated by the letters Wk. However, don't be bound by any of the categories you find the recipes in; there is absolutely no reason why you can't have a lunch dish as your main meal or breakfast dish for lunch – just as long as you have the correct number of servings of protein, fat, vegetables and so on for the day.

BREAKFASTS

Mixed Berry Bruschetta

Serves 2

Berries are a great source of vitamin C and the cancer-protective phytochemical ellagic acid. Each serving provides 45 per cent of the calcium and 20 per cent of the folic acid the body needs each day.

200 g/7 oz mixed berries, such as strawberries, blueberries and
blackberries
2 slices crusty mixed-grain bread
1 tsp olive oil spread
$^1/_2$ tsp cinnamon
6 tbsp low fat natural yoghurt
or fromage frais

Wash, hull and dry the berries.

Lightly toast the bread on both sides then scrape a little of the spread over each slice.

Place a handful of the berries on the two toasted slices of bread. Sprinkle some cinnamon on top and serve accompanied by 3 spoonfuls of yoghurt.

Nutritional info per serving
1 fruit portion, 1 starchy food portion, 1 dairy portion
Calories 200 kcal/835 kJ; Fat 2.4 g (monounsaturated 0.8 g, polyunsaturated 0.6 g,
saturated 1 g); Protein 10 g; Carbohydrate 35 g; Fibre: 4 g; Salt: 0.7 g

Fresh Bircher Muesli with Fruit and Maple Syrup

Serves 2

Oats are a great filling breakfast, as their slow-release starch keeps hunger at bay.

The Brazil nuts boost the selenium and zinc in this recipe –

each serving provides 40 per cent of the selenium and a third of the zinc we need each day.

130 g/4½ oz rolled oats
80 ml/3 fl oz red grape juice
2 tbsp low fat natural yoghurt
1 ripe banana, 2 fresh figs or a peeled and grated apple
    or pear
2 tbsp chopped and toasted Brazil nuts
2 tsp maple syrup or honey (optional)

Place the oats in a small bowl, cover with the grape juice and soak overnight to soften the oats.

When you are ready to serve, add the yoghurt. Spoon the oats into breakfast bowls and top with sliced banana or quartered figs. Sprinkle with the chopped Brazil nuts and drizzle with maple syrup or honey if required.

Nutritional info per serving
2 starchy food portions, 1 fruit portion, 1 fat portion, ½ dairy food portion
Calories 400 kcal/1672 kJ; Fat: 13 g (monounsaturated 5 g, polyunsaturated 5 g, saturated 3 g); Protein 10 g; Carbohydrate 60 g; Fibre 4 g; Salt 0.1 g

Couscous with Apricots and Mango

Serves 2

You may not have thought of having couscous for breakfast but it is a filling and delicious way to start the day.

Dried apricots are a great source of iron while vitamin C-rich mango helps make sure you absorb the iron from these.

100 g/3½ oz couscous
250 ml/8 fl oz semi-skimmed milk
1 vanilla bean, split
100 g/3½ oz dried apricots, chopped
100 g/3½ oz fresh mango, cut into cubes

Place the couscous and milk in a large saucepan and bring to the boil. Scrape the seeds from the vanilla bean into the saucepan. Reduce the heat and simmer for about 5 minutes until the couscous is soft. Drain, reserving the hot milk. Set the couscous aside in a warm place.

Place the apricots in the hot milk and leave to soak until they become plump.

Place the couscous in bowls and add the apricots, fresh mango and some of the vanilla milk. Serve hot or warm.

Nutritional info per serving
2 starchy food portions, 1/2 dairy portion, 2 fruit portions
Calories 290 kcal/1212 kJ; Fat 3 g (monounsaturated 0.5 g, polyunsaturated 1 g, saturated 1.5 g); Protein 10 g; Carbohydrate 60 g; Fibre 5 g; Salt 0.2 g

Granola

Makes 4 servings
The whole grains, berries and nuts in this recipe are packed with cancer-protective fibre and phytochemicals. Each serving provides 20 per cent of the selenium we need each day.

1 tbsp sunflower oil
1/2 tbsp clear honey
1/2 tbsp lemon juice
115 g/4 oz large rolled oats
30 g/1 oz wheat flakes
15 g/1/2 oz sesame seeds
20 g/3/4 oz pecans, finely chopped
20 g/3/4 oz Brazil nuts, finely chopped
30 g/1 oz sultanas
30 g/1 oz dried mango, chopped
30 g/1 oz dried blueberries

Preheat the oven to 140°C/275°F/gas 1.

Place the oil, honey and lemon juice in a pan, and stir over a gentle heat until melted and evenly mixed, without letting it boil.

Remove from the heat and add all the remaining ingredients except for the sultanas, dried mango and blueberries. Stir and mix until evenly coated.

Spread the mixture on two baking sheets lined with non-stick baking parchment. Bake in the preheated oven for an hour, stirring frequently, until crisp and golden brown.

Allow the granola to cool, stirring occasionally to break up any lumps. Mix with the sultanas, mango and blueberries and store in an airtight container.

Granola is delicious served with milk or yoghurt and fresh fruit. It also makes a good crunchy snack.

Nutritional info per serving
1 starchy food portion, 1 fruit portion, 1 fat portion
Calories 300 kcal/1254 kJ; Fat 14 g (monounsaturated 7 g, polyunsaturated 5 g, saturated 2 g); Protein 7 g; Carbohydrate 35 g; Fibre 7 g; Salt 0.06 g

Fromage Frais Pancakes with Honey and Blueberries

Serves 2
Each serving of these tasty pancakes provides 20 per cent of the calcium and 40 per cent of the folic acid we need each day. The berries add a lovely flavour and are a great source of phytochemicals.

PANCAKE BATTER
40 g/1¼ oz plain flour
40 g/1¼ oz wholemeal flour
80 ml/3 fl oz warm milk
1 tsp sugar
¼ tsp salt
1 egg, separated
5 g dry yeast
½ tbsp fromage frais
1 tsp olive oil spread (for cooking)

TOPPING

1 tbsp Acacia honey

150 g/5^1/$_2$ oz blueberries

3 tbsp low fat fromage frais or yoghurt

Place the flours in a large mixing bowl and make a well in the centre. Add the warm milk, sugar and salt, and mix well. Stir in the egg yolk and add the yeast. Mix well until you have a smooth batter. Cover and leave in a warm place for about an hour, until the batter has doubled in size.

Whisk the egg white until it resembles soft peaks. Fold it into the pancake batter. Stir in the fromage frais.

Place a heavy, non-stick frying pan, about 18 cm/7 inches in diameter, on a medium-high heat. With a pastry brush, brush the surface with a little olive oil spread. Ladle spoonfuls of the pancake mixture into the pan and cook until golden brown on each side. Allow the pancakes to cook for about 40 seconds on each side.

Serve hot with the honey, blueberries and low fat fromage frais or yoghurt.

Nutritional info per serving
1 starchy food portion, 1 fruit portion, ½ dairy portion
Calories 300 kcal/1254 kJ; Fat 8 g (monounsaturated 3.5 g, polyunsaturated 2 g, saturated 2.5 g); Protein 15 g; Carbohydrate 40 g; Fibre 4 g; Salt 0.25 g

Cabbage, Turkey and Bacon Soup

Serves 4

This hearty winter soup is packed with protein and fibre. Cabbage is a great source of the phytochemical indole-3-carbinol, as well as folic acid and vitamin C.

1 tbsp olive oil
2 onions, sliced
4 rashers lean bacon, trimmed of fat
200 g/7 oz turkey breast, chopped
4 carrots, chopped
1 kg/2¼ lb green cabbage, washed and thinly shredded
1 litre/1¾ pints chicken stock (made with ½ stock cube)
freshly ground pepper

Heat the olive oil in a large saucepan, add the onion, bacon and turkey and brown lightly. Add the carrots, cabbage and stock, bring to the boil, reduce the heat and simmer for 45–60 minutes. Season to taste with pepper. Serve with wholemeal bread.

Nutritional info per serving
2 ½ protein portions, 3 vegetable portions
Calories 250 kcal/1045 kJ; Fat 9 g (monounsaturated 4 g, polyunsaturated 2.5 g, saturated 2.5 g); Protein 20 g; Carbohydrate 25 g; Fibre 9 g; Salt 1.25 g

Lentil and Mushroom Soup

Serves 4

This delicious soup combines the goodness of lentils (which contain iron, magnesium, calcium, selenium and folic acid) with phytochemical-rich mushrooms. Each serving contains 75 per cent of your daily iron requirement so make sure you have some fruit or fruit juice with the soup, as this will ensure you absorb the iron.

2 tbsp extra virgin olive oil
1 carrot, finely chopped
2 celery stalks, finely chopped
1 onion, finely chopped
1 leek, finely chopped
100 g/3½ oz mushrooms
200 g/7 oz brown lentils, soaked overnight
3 rosemary sprigs, chopped
small bunch thyme, leaves only, chopped
750 ml/27 fl oz vegetable stock
2 tsp red wine vinegar
small bunch flat-leafed parsley, chopped
freshly ground pepper

Heat the olive oil in a large saucepan over medium-low heat. Add the chopped vegetables, cover and cook gently for about 5 minutes until translucent.

Drain the lentils and add to the vegetables. Cook for 3 minutes, stirring. Add the rosemary and thyme to the pan along with the vegetable stock.

Bring the soup to the boil, reduce the heat and simmer over a medium heat for 1 hour, until the lentils are very soft, skimming away any impurities which rise to the top.

Purée the soup in a food processor or blender, pour it back into the pan, add the vinegar and season with pepper. Bring back almost to the boil. Add the parsley and serve with wholemeal bread.

Nutritional info per serving
1 protein portion, 1 ½ vegetable portions
Calories 210 kcal/878 kJ; Fat 5 g (monounsaturated 3 g, polyunsaturated 2 g, saturated 0 g); Protein 25 g; Carbohydrate 30 g; Fibre 7 g; Salt 1 g

Root Vegetable Soup

Serves 4

This golden soup is one of my recipes. It's simply bursting with carotenoids, one of the bioactive components of food which play a part in reducing breast cancer risk.

1 large onion

1 tbsp olive oil

1 tsp sesame oil

2 large carrots

$^1/_2$ medium-sized swede

2 turnips

1 small-medium sweet potato

2 parsnips

150 ml/5 fl oz fresh orange juice

600 ml/1 pint vegetable stock (made with stock cube)

fresh rosemary

freshly ground pepper

Chop the onion fairly finely and fry in the olive and sesame oil until softened.

Meanwhile, peel the remaining vegetables and chop into 2 cm/3/4 inch chunks. Add to the onion, and gently fry for another few minutes, stirring regularly.

Add the orange juice, then the stock and some chopped fresh rosemary. Season with pepper. Bring to the boil and simmer gently for 30 minutes.

Allow to cool for at least 10 minutes then liquidize. Reheat before serving, but do not allow the soup to boil. Serve with wholemeal bread.

Nutritional info per serving

2 vegetable portions, $^1/_2$ starchy food portion

Calories 150 kcal/627 kJ; Fat 5 g (monounsaturated 3 g, polyunsaturated 1 g, saturated 1 g); Protein 2 g; Carbohydrate 25 g; Fibre 5 g; Salt 0.5 g

Asparagus and Avocado Soup

Serves 4

This soup is quick, simple to prepare – perfect when asparagus is in season.

All the ingredients used in this soup are uncooked to retain the maximum nutrient content. It is packed with beta-carotene and vitamin E and has the added advantage of being simple and quick to prepare. It is served cold so it is ideal for warm weather.

2 bunches asparagus, trimmed and chopped
1 avocado, peeled and chopped
a handful of fresh basil leaves
2 tbsp lemon juice
grated zest of 1 lemon
2 tbsp extra virgin olive oil
1 small onion, peeled and grated
pinch of salt and freshly ground pepper

Place the asparagus, avocado, basil leaves, lemon juice and zest, oil, onion and 300 ml/10 fl oz water in a food processor and purée until smooth. Season to taste and strain through a fine sieve. Serve cold.

Nutritional info per serving
1 vegetable portion, 1 fat portion
Calories 140 kcal/585 kJ; Fat 10 g (monounsaturated 7 g, polyunsaturated 1 g, saturated 2 g); Protein 5 g; Carbohydrate 5 g; Fibre 4 g; Salt 1 g

Marinated Mackerel with Cucumber and Dill Salad

Serves 4

This dish needs to marinade so it has to be prepared in advance. Canned mackerel is fantastic value and a very good source of omega-3 fats, vitamin D and selenium.

200 g/7 oz mackerel fillets in oil, drained
60 ml/2 fl oz white wine vinegar
8 black peppercorns, crushed
2 bay leaves
2 cloves, crushed
4 allspice berries, crushed
¼ tsp yellow mustard seeds
1 shallot, finely chopped
1 tsp small capers, chopped
1 tbsp chopped rosemary
1 tbsp chopped thyme

SALAD
1 large cucumber
pinch of salt
100 ml/3½ fl oz fromage frais
juice of ½ lemon
2 tbsp finely chopped dill

Drain the mackerel fillets and set aside. Mix together the vinegar, peppercorns, bay leaves, cloves, allspice berries, mustard seeds, shallot, capers, rosemary and thyme.

Place the mackerel fillets in a large shallow dish and cover with the marinade. Cover the dish and refrigerate for 4–6 hours.

Begin preparing the salad 30 minutes before you wish to serve it. The secret of this salad is to peel the cucumber and cut it into very thin slices. Place the slices in a sieve, sprinkle with a pinch of salt and leave for 30 minutes or so to drain. Rinse the excess salt from the cucumber slices and dry them. Place the slices in a medium bowl with the fromage frais, lemon juice and dill, and mix well. Serve at once with the marinated mackerel and some wholemeal bread.

Nutritional info per serving
2 protein portions, 1 vegetable portion
Calories 180 kcal/752 kJ; Fat 12 g (monounsaturated 5 g, polyunsaturated 4 g, saturated 3 g); Protein 11 g; Carbohydrate 3 g; Fibre 1 g; Salt 1 g

Griddled Sardines with Tomato, Avocado and Lime Salsa

Serves 4

Sardines are wonderful fish – they're packed with goodness, have a great flavour and are excellent value. Unfortunately, many people, whilst happy to eat them when holidaying in the Mediterranean, are reluctant to cook them at home. If you don't like preparing fish, then get your fishmonger to scale and fillet the sardines for you. Simply make sure the fish you choose have a fresh, shiny and silver-blue skin, are firm to the touch, and that the eye looks bright.

This dish is a great combination of the cancer-protective goodness of oily fish and carotenoid-rich tomatoes.

16 sardines
1 tbsp extra virgin olive oil

SALSA
3 large tomatoes
1 large avocado, stoned and peeled
1 red onion, finely chopped
1 garlic clove, finely chopped
1 small red chilli, seeded and chopped
5 tbsp chopped coriander
4 tbsp green olives, pitted and chopped
juice of 1 lime
salt and freshly ground pepper

Make the salsa first. Pour boiling water over the tomatoes and leave for a minute or so. Drain off the water, allow the tomatoes to cool, peel the skins off, cut the tomatoes in half and remove the seeds. Cut the flesh of the tomatoes and the avocado into small squares. Place in a bowl and add the onion, garlic, chilli, coriander, olives and lime juice. Season and add more lime juice if required. Mix well and set aside.

If your fish are not ready-prepared, cut off the heads and remove the backbones. This is done by making cuts along both sides of the backbone, all along its length, then carefully taking out the bone and as many of the fine bones as you can (alternatively just remove the head – sardines are small enough that they can be eaten whole).

Place a heavy griddle pan or ridged chargrill pan on high heat and when really hot, brush with the olive oil. Add the sardine fillets and cook for about 2 minutes on each side.

Divide the tomato and avocado salsa between four plates and top with 4 sardine fillets. Serve with an additional portion of green salad.

Nutritional info per serving
2 protein portions, 1 fat portion, 1 vegetable portion
Calories 250 kcal/1045 kJ; Fat 19 g (monounsaturated 10 g, polyunsaturated 5 g, saturated 4 g); Protein 13 g; Carbohydrate 8 g; Fibre 4 g; Salt 1 g

Warm King Prawn and Endive Salad with Grapefruit and Peanuts

Serves 4

This innovative combination of flavours produces a luxurious, crisp and very citrusy salad that is packed with goodness. The prawns are a good source of selenium and magnesium, the pink grapefruit provides lycopene, and the peanuts contain resveraterol, monounsaturated fat and magnesium.

2 medium grapefruits (preferably pink), peeled and segmented
200 g/7 oz green curly endive leaves, washed
1 red onion, sliced
2 tsp extra virgin olive oil
12 king prawns, peeled, tail left intact or 150 g/5^1/$_2$ oz peeled prawns
salt and freshly ground pepper
40 g/1^1/$_2$ oz shelled peanuts, coarsely chopped

SHALLOT AND CORIANDER VINAIGRETTE

1½ tbsp extra virgin olive oil

1 medium shallot, grated

2 tbsp red wine vinegar

1 tbsp finely chopped coriander

Combine the grapefruit segments, endive leaves and red onion in a salad bowl.

Heat the olive oil in a heavy-based pan and, when very hot, add the king prawns and cook for about 2 minutes on each side, until brown. Season with salt and pepper and keep warm.

To make the vinaigrette, combine all the ingredients, season with salt and pepper, and mix well.

Divide the salad between four plates, sprinkle with the peanuts, top each portion with three king prawns, and drizzle with the dressing.

Nutritional info per serving
1 protein portion, 1 vegetable portion, 2 fat portions
Calories 180 kcal/752 kJ; Fat 11 g (monounsaturated 7 g, polyunsaturated 2 g, saturated 2 g); Protein 13 g; Carbohydrate 14 g; Fibre 4 g; Salt 1.5 g

Pasta with Fresh Tomato Sauce

Serves 4

This simple pasta dish is filling, tasty and quick to make. If you wish to add some protein simply stir in your favourite canned fish or some cooked chicken or turkey.

The tomatoes are a great source of folic acid, vitamin C and the carotenoid lycopene.

4 tsp extra virgin olive oil

4 garlic cloves, crushed

20 ripe medium-sized tomatoes,
    roughly chopped

½ tsp sweet paprika

200 g/7 oz dried pasta
2 tbsp balsamic vinegar
large bunch of basil, roughly torn
salt and freshly ground pepper

Pour the olive oil into a large saucepan. Add the garlic and heat briefly (do not let it brown). Add the tomatoes and paprika to the pan and cook for 10–12 minutes.

Meanwhile, cook the pasta in a pan of boiling salted water for approximately 7–8 minutes. Drain the pasta.

Add the balsamic vinegar, basil leaves, seasoning and pasta to the sauce; mix well and serve immediately.

Nutritional info per serving
2 starchy food portions, 2 vegetable portions, 1 fat portion
Calories 270 kcal/1129 kJ; Fat 5 g (monounsaturated 3 g, polyunsaturated 1 g, saturated 1 g); Protein 8 g; Carbohydrate 50 g; Fibre 8 g; Salt 0.1 g

Pearl Barley 'Risotto' with Crab and Chilli

Serves 4

Pearl barley is the basis for this delicious low-calorie risotto. The dish is a great source of magnesium, zinc, selenium and folic acid. Serve it with steamed green vegetables or fresh salad.

260 g/9 oz crab meat (fresh or canned)
2 tsp extra virgin olive oil
2 shallots, finely chopped
1 garlic clove, finely chopped
$^1/_2$ tsp chilli flakes
200 g/7 oz pearl barley
1 litre/1$^3/_4$ pt hot chicken stock
freshly ground pepper

If the crab meat is canned, rinse it and set it aside to drain.

Heat the olive oil in a large saucepan, add the shallots, garlic and chilli flakes, and sauté until the shallots are translucent.

Add the barley and stir until well coated with oil. Increase the heat and start adding small ladlefuls of hot stock, bringing to the boil. Reduce the heat to very low and simmer, stirring constantly, adding more stock as the previous addition is absorbed (just like a risotto). Cook until the barley is soft, about 10–12 minutes.

Add the crab meat to the pan and simmer for a further 2–3 minutes. Season to taste and serve hot.

Nutritional info per serving
2 protein portions, 2 starchy food portions
Calories 300 kcal/1254 kJ; Fat 8 g (monounsaturated 4 g, polyunsaturated 3 g, saturated 1 g); Protein 17 g; Carbohydrate 40 g; Fibre 5 g; Salt 1.4 g

Tuna with Beans

Serves 4
This simple, low-calorie salad combines the goodness of tuna, white beans and tomatoes. Each portion provides half of the daily requirement for vitamin D, vitamin E and iron, and all the daily requirement for selenium.

200 g/7 oz dried white beans (or use 400 g/14 oz can
    precooked beans)
2 garlic cloves, roughly chopped
salt and freshly ground pepper
1 red onion, very finely sliced
350 g/12 oz fresh tomatoes, finely chopped
2 tbsp extra virgin olive oil
4 tbsp finely chopped parsley
400 g/14 oz can tuna in brine

Soak the dried beans overnight in cold water. Rinse, transfer to a saucepan, top up with cold water and bring to the boil. Add the garlic, season, cover, and simmer for 1–1½ hours or until beans are cooked. (If using canned beans, just rinse them well, add the rest of the ingredients and serve.)

Strain, and place the beans in a serving dish. Add the onion and tomato, season to taste, then add the olive oil. Mix together and chill.

When ready to serve, add the tuna and parsley and mix thoroughly.

Nutritional info per serving
2 protein portions, 2 vegetable portions, 1 fat portion
Calories 450 kcal/1881 kJ; Fat 9 g (monounsaturated 6 g, polyunsaturated 1.5 g, saturated 1.5 g); Protein 40 g; Carbohydrate 50 g; Fibre 15 g; Salt 1.8 g

SALADS AND SIDE DISHES

Baby Potato, Blood Orange and Asparagus Salad

Serves 4

Walnuts are a great source of omega-3 fats, asparagus is rich in folic acid and oranges are a good source of calcium and vitamin C – the combination also tastes delicious!

200 g/7 oz baby potatoes, cleaned
12 thin green asparagus stalks, peeled
salt and freshly ground pepper
100 g/3½ oz beetroot salad leaves or Swiss chard, washed and dried
2 small blood oranges, peeled and thinly sliced
4 tbsp shelled walnuts, lightly toasted

WALNUT VINAIGRETTE
1 tbsp red wine vinegar
1 tbsp walnut oil
2 tbsp olive oil

Boil the baby potatoes for 20 minutes until cooked; drain and cool. Cook the asparagus in boiling salted water, but very briefly so it keeps its colour and crispy texture.

To make the walnut vinaigrette, whisk together the vinegar, walnut and olive oils. Season to taste.

Toss the beet salad leaves in the vinaigrette and place on the centre of each plate. Arrange the potatoes, asparagus and blood orange slices on top. Sprinkle with the walnuts.

Nutritional info per serving
½ fruit portion, 1 vegetable portion, 1 fat portion
Calories 225 kcal/940 kJ; Fat 13 g (monounsaturated 4 g, polyunsaturated 8 g, saturated 1 g); Protein 6 g; Carbohydrate 20 g; Fibre 4 g; Salt 0.1 g

Sicilian Salad of Fennel and Oranges

Serves 4

Fennel goes well with citrus flavours such as orange. In this recipe it is used raw but it is also lovely sautéed, baked or braised. Look for fennel that has a tight head, crisp stalks and no brown spots on the white ribs.

This tasty salad is rich in folic acid, magnesium and vitamin C.

2 large oranges
1 large fennel bulb
2 tbsp olive oil
1 tbsp lemon juice
freshly ground pepper
200 g/7 oz fresh wild rocket leaves
40 g/1¼ oz pine nuts, toasted
4 anchovy fillets

Peel the oranges with a very sharp knife and slice into rounds. Place in a bowl.

Trim the base from the fennel, cut away the leaves then slice very thinly. Add the fennel to the oranges, and add the olive oil, lemon juice and pepper to taste. Mix well, leave for 5–6 minutes then toss with the rocket leaves.

Sprinkle with the pine nuts, decorate with the anchovies, and serve.

Nutritional info per serving
½ fruit portion, 1 vegetable portion, 1 fat portion
Calories 190 kcal/794 kJ; Fat 13 g (monounsaturated 7 g, polyunsaturated 5 g, saturated 1 g); Protein 5 g; Carbohydrate 10 g; Fibre 3 g; Salt 0.7 g

Pink Grapefruit Salad with Radishes

Serves 4

Pink grapefruits are rich in folic acid, vitamin C and lycopene.

1 pink grapefruit, cut into segments
1 cucumber, peeled and grated
2 medium apples, peeled and grated
2 celery sticks, finely diced
3 spring onions, finely chopped
5 radishes, washed and grated
2 tbsp finely chopped fresh parsley
juice from 2 pink grapefruits and 1 orange

Combine the fruits, vegetables and parsley in a bowl, pour on the grapefruit and orange juice and chill before serving.

Nutritional info per serving
1¹/₂ fruit portions, 1 vegetable portion
Calories 90 kcal/376 kJ; Fat 0 g; Protein 2 g; Carbohydrate 20 g; Fibre 3 g; Salt 0.06 g

Bulgur Wheat, Chickpea and Grape Salad

Serves 4

The bulgur wheat and chickpeas make this a filling fibre-, protein- and magnesium-rich salad – and the grapes are, of course, full of the phytochemical reseveraterol.

150 g/5¹/₂ oz bulgur wheat
2 tsp extra virgin olive oil
juice and zest from 4 lemons
400 g/14 oz can chickpeas, drained
1 large red onion, peeled and finely chopped
100 g/3¹/₂ oz grated carrots
200 g/7 oz seedless green grapes, halved
1 bunch fresh basil, finely chopped

Place the bulgur a saucepan, cover with water and simmer until soft. Drain and leave to cool.

Once cooled, place the bulgur in a large bowl and add the oil, lemon juice and zest. Mix well and add the chickpeas, onion, carrots, grapes and basil. Mix gently and serve.

Nutritional info per serving
1 protein portion, 1 starchy food portion, 1 fruit portion
Calories 250 kcal/1045 kJ; Fat 5.5 g (monounsaturated 2.5 g, polyunsaturated 1.5 g, saturated 1.5 g); Protein 8 g; Carbohydrate 40 g; Fibre 4 g; Salt 0.4 g

Couscous Salad with Grapes and Pistachio Nuts

Serves 4

This light and fluffy salad has an unusual but delicious mixture of flavours and textures.

The vegetables, fruits and herbs are packed with phytochemicals, as well as folic acid, vitamin C and beta-carotene, while the pistachio nuts are a great source of monounsaturated fats.

200 g/7 oz couscous
2 large ripe tomatoes, finely diced
$^1/_2$ green pepper (capsicum), seeded and chopped
$^1/_2$ cucumber, peeled and finely sliced
80–100 g/2$^1/_2$–3$^1/_2$ oz seedless red grapes, halved
    or 30 g/1 oz raisins
1 small garlic clove, crushed
salt and freshly ground pepper
2 tsp olive oil
juice of 1 lemon
5 tbsp chopped parsley
5 tbsp chopped chives
3 tbsp chopped mint
4 tbsp pistachio nuts, roughly chopped and lightly toasted

Place the couscous in a bowl, cover with hot water, cover the bowl and leave to soak until soft, about 5 minutes. Drain if necessary and keep aside.

In a large bowl, mix together the tomatoes, green pepper, cucumber, grapes and garlic. Add the couscous and mix well. Season with salt and pepper, then add the olive oil and lemon juice, and finally mix in the parsley and mint.

Chill the salad for about 2 hours. Sprinkle with the pistachios just before serving.

Nutritional info per serving
2 starchy food portions, 1 fat portion, 1 vegetable portion, ½ fruit portion
Calories 270 kcal/1129 kJ; Fat 12 g (monounsaturated 6.5 g, polyunsaturated 3.5 g, saturated 2 g); Protein 6 g; Carbohydrate 35 g; Fibre 3 g; Salt 0.2 g

Roasted Root Vegetables and Broccoli

Serves 4
This tasty combination of root vegetables and broccoli is packed with phytochemicals.

4 tsp olive oil
600 g/1 lb 5 oz root vegetables (potato, swede, turnip, carrot, parsnip) cut into chunks
200 g/7 oz broccoli
salt and freshly ground pepper
small bunch of parsley, finely chopped

Preheat the oven to 200°/C/400°F/gas 6.

Heat the oil in a roasting dish on the stove. Add the vegetables and cook for 5–6 minutes over a high heat, until they start to colour, turning occasionally. Season to taste and add enough water to cover the bottom of the dish. Reheat to boiling and reduce the liquid, about 4–5 minutes.

Place the dish in the oven and cook for about 20 minutes, by which time the water should have evaporated. Turn the vegetables and cook for a further 5 minutes to add colour. Sprinkle with parsley to serve.

Nutritional info per serving
2 vegetable portions, 1 fat portion
Calories 90 kcal/376 kJ; Fat 5 g (monounsaturated 3 g, polyunsaturated 1 g, saturated 1 g); Protein 2 g; Carbohydrate 6 g; Fibre 4 g; Salt 0 g

Carrot Gratin

Serves 4

This is a rather elegant way of preparing any kind of root vegetable. It combines the goodness of root vegetables (which contain carotenoids, folic acid and magnesium) with fromage frais (which provides calcium). Each serving provides 25 per cent of the calcium and 20 per cent of the folic acid and magnesium we need.

1 tbsp olive oil
2 shallots, finely chopped
600 g/1 lb 5 oz carrots, grated
2 apples, grated
40 g/1¼ oz golden sultanas
200 g/7 oz fromage frais
2 large egg yolks, beaten
1 tsp honey
¼ tsp ground coriander
½ tsp ground cumin
salt and freshly ground pepper
150 g/5½ oz wholemeal breadcrumbs

Preheat the oven to 180°C/350°F/gas 4.

Heat the oil in a large non-stick pan, add the shallots and cook until soft. Add the carrots, apple and sultanas; continue cooking for another 5–7 minutes, stirring all the time.

Lightly oil a medium baking dish and pour in the apple mixture.

In a mixing bowl, mix the fromage frais and egg yolks then add the honey, coriander and cumin. Season with salt and pepper. Pour the mixture over the carrots in the baking dish.

In a small frying pan brown the breadcrumbs for about 2 minutes. Sprinkle on top of the carrot and fromage frais mixture and bake for about 25–30 minutes until golden brown.

Nutritional info per serving
2 vegetable portions, 1 fruit portion, 2 starchy food portions, ½ dairy portion
Calories 300 kcal/1254 kJ; Fat 11 g (monounsaturated 4 g, polyunsaturated 3 g, saturated 4 g); Protein 10 g; Carbohydrate 40 g; Fibre 7 g; Salt 0.7 g

Chargrilled Vegetable Salad

Serves 4

This recipe is a good source of vitamin C, folic acid and beta-carotene – it's also delicious!

500 g/1 lb 2 oz aubergines (eggplants), cut into 3 cm/1¼ in slices
4 courgettes (zucchini), cut into 3 cm/1¼ in slices
1 green pepper (capsicum), cut into 2 cm/¾ in slices
1 yellow pepper (capsicum), cut into 2 cm/¾ in slices
6 plum tomatoes, halved lengthways

DRESSING
4 tsp extra virgin olive oil
1 tbsp balsamic vinegar
3 garlic cloves, crushed
small bunch basil, roughly chopped

Place a ridged chargrill pan on high heat and when really hot, add the aubergines and courgette slices a few at a time. Cook for 3–5 minutes, turning to cooked evenly. Repeat with all the slices.

Chargrill the peppers for 2–3 minutes, turning so they are evenly cooked. Now cook the tomatoes, skin side first. Place all the vegetables together in a large bowl and leave to cool.

Mix together the dressing ingredients, pour over the vegetables, season to taste and serve as required.

Nutritional info per serving
4 vegetable portions, 1 fat portion
Calories 200 kcal/836 kJ; Fat 14 g (monounsaturated 10 g, polyunsaturated 2 g, saturated 2 g); Protein 5 g; Carbohydrate 15 g; Fibre 7 g; Salt 0 g

Chargrilled Broccoli, Fennel and Radicchio

Serves 4

This is a good source of vitamin C, folic acid and beta-carotene. It's particularly good served with pasta or tomato-based dishes.

1 head fennel
2 heads radicchio
16 broccoli florets
4 tsp extra virgin olive oil
1 tsp balsamic vinegar
juice of 1 lemon
salt and freshly ground pepper

Trim the fennel and radicchio and cut into quarters lengthways. Heat a griddle or ridged chargrill pan. (If you do not have a griddle or chargrill pan, then use a heavy bottomed frying pan instead to dry fry the vegetables.)

Add the fennel, cook for 2 minutes, turning when brown, then add broccoli and cook the same way. Now add the radicchio and continue to cook for a further 2 minutes or until the leaves start to soften. Remove to a serving dish and leave to cool.

Mix together the oil, vinegar and lemon juice, and season to taste. Pour over the griddled vegetables and serve.

Nutritional info per serving
3 vegetable portions, 1 fat portion
Calories 180 kcal/752 kJ; Fat 7 g (monounsaturated 5 g, polyunsaturated 1 g, saturated 1 g); Protein 7 g; Carbohydrate 5 g; Fibre 7 g; Salt 0.2 g

VEGETARIAN DISHES

Sweet Potato and Cream Cheese Pancakes
Serves 2
These delicious pancakes combine the goodness of low fat dairy products with carotenoid-rich sweet potatoes and the phytochemical carnesol in sage.

250 g/9 oz sweet potatoes
80 g/2¹/₂ oz low fat cream cheese
1 egg
20 g/³/₄ oz plain flour or potato flour if preferred
¹/₂ onion, finely chopped
2 tbsp finely chopped sage
salt and freshly ground pepper
1 tbsp olive oil

Peel and grate the potatoes. Squeeze any excess moisture from the potatoes and place in a bowl. Add the cheese, egg, flour, onion and sage. Season with salt and pepper and mix well. Shape small patties, using your hands, and set aside until ready to cook.

Heat the oil in a large non-stick frying pan over medium heat, add the patties and fry for about 3 minutes on each side, until golden in colour. Serve with a bowl of freshly prepared mixed salad.

Nutritional info per serving
1 dairy portion, 2 starchy food portions, 1 fat portion
Calories 300 kcal/1254 kJ; Fat 13 g (monounsaturated 7 g, polyunsaturated 2 g, saturated 4 g); Protein 12 g; Carbohydrate 35 g; Fibre 4 g; Salt 0.7 g

Pumpkin, Chickpea and Coriander Curry

Serves 4

If you're not a fan of pumpkin, courgettes (zucchini) can be used just as successfully in this curry. It's quick to prepare and tastes creamy – but it's low in calories and healthy, too.

800 g/1³/₄ lb pumpkin or courgettes (zucchini)
2 tbsp extra virgin olive oil
¹/₂ tsp ready-made green curry paste
6 spring onions, washed and sliced
3 garlic cloves, crushed
1 red chilli, chopped finely
100 g/3¹/₂ oz cooked chickpeas
1 tbsp fennel seeds
100 ml/3¹/₂ fl oz vegetable stock
100 ml/3¹/₂ fl oz coconut milk
small bunch coriander, washed and finely chopped
 4 tbsp low fat natural yoghurt
 pinch of salt and freshly ground pepper

Peel the pumpkin or courgettes and cut into 2 cm/³/₄ in pieces. Place the oil in a large sauté pan, add the pumpkin or courgettes pieces and sauté, together with the curry paste, until slightly browned around the edges.

Stirring well, add the spring onions, garlic, chilli, chickpeas, fennel seeds, stock and coconut milk. Simmer for 20 minutes until the curry is almost cooked and sauce had thickened and reduced. Season to taste.

Sprinkle with the coriander and serve with a few tablespoons of natural yoghurt. A mixed salad and boiled rice or chapatti make good accompaniments.

Nutritional info per serving
¹/₂ protein portion, 1 dairy portion, 2 vegetable portions
Calories 150 kcal/627 kJ; Fat 8 g (monounsaturated 5 g, polyunsaturated 2 g, saturated 1 g); Protein 6 g; Carbohydrate 10 g; Fibre 4 g; Salt 0.6 g

Napoleon of Aubergines with Celeriac and Feta Cheese

Serves 4

This delicious recipe is very easy to prepare at home. The aubergine provides beta-carotene while the celeriac is a great source of calcium, magnesium and folic acid.

2 small aubergines (eggplants)
pinch of salt and freshly ground pepper
1 tbsp flour
4 tsp extra virgin olive oil
500 g/1 lb 2 oz cooked celeriac, roughly chopped
2 tbsp fresh oregano leaves, chopped finely
120 g/4 oz feta cheese, roughly chopped

Trim, wash and dry the aubergines. Cut lengthways into 5 mm/1/4 in slices. Season and coat with flour.

Heat the oil in a non-stick shallow frying pan and gently fry each slice on both sides until lightly browned. Drain on kitchen paper.

Preheat the oven to 200°C/400°F/gas 6.

Place the cooked celeriac, oregano and cheese in a medium pan and heat, stirring them together, for just few minutes.

Starting with the largest of the aubergine slices, assemble on a baking sheet, four piles of aubergine, inter-layered with the celeriac-cheese mixture, finishing each pile with the smallest of the slices. Bake in the preheated oven for 5 minutes. Serve hot

Nutritional info per serving
1 dairy portion, 3 vegetable portions, 1/2 fat portion
Calories 180 kcal/752 kJ; Fat 12 g (monounsaturated 5 g, polyunsaturated 2 g, saturated 5 g); Protein 8 g; Carbohydrate 10 g; Fibre 7 g; Salt 1.5 g

Oyster Mushrooms in Ginger Sauce with Colcannon

Serves 4

This delicious low-calorie recipe is packed with phytochemicals. Oyster mushrooms, with their subtle, delicate flavour, cook beautifully and combine to stunning effect with the ginger sauce and pak choi colcannon.

300 g/10^1/2 oz fresh oyster mushrooms, cleaned
1 tbsp grated ginger
2 garlic cloves, crushed
10 g/^{1}/3 oz olive oil spread

PAK CHOI COLCANNON
600 g/1 lb 5 oz potatoes, boiled in salted water
10 g/^{1}/3 oz olive oil spread
5 tbsp milk
100 g/3^1/2 oz tofu, cut into small cubes
200 g/7 oz pak choi (bok choy), cleaned and lightly blanched
1 bunch spring onions, thinly sliced
2 tbsp finely chopped parsley
salt and freshly ground pepper

First, make the colcannon. Drain the potatoes and, while hot, mash in the olive oil spread and milk until creamy. Sauté the tofu until golden brown and crispy. Place the crispy tofu, pak choi, spring onion and parsley in a large bowl and mix well. Fold them through the potato purée and season to taste. Keep the colcannon warm.

Mix the ginger with a little of the olive oil spread and set aside. Melt the rest of the olive oil spread in a shallow pan. Add the mushrooms to it, turning them now and again, until lightly browned. Now add the garlic, and cook for a further 4 minutes. Now add the ginger mixture and take the pan off the heat immediately.

To serve: spoon some colcannon in the middle of each plate and place some of the gingered oyster mushroom on top. Drizzle the pan sauces around. Serve with salad steamed vegetables.

Nutritional info per serving
½ protein portion, 1/2 dairy portion, 2 vegetable portions, 2 starchy food portions
Calories 200 kcal/836 kJ; Fat 5 g (monounsaturated 2 g, polyunsaturated 2 g, saturated 1 g); Protein 8 g; Carbohydrate 30 g; Fibre 3 g; Salt 0.5 g

Roast Pepper Parcels with Spinach, Hazelnuts and Cottage Cheese

Serves 4

Cooking peppers over a direct flame or on top of an electric hob gives them a slightly smoky flavour but it does not lead to the formation of harmful chemicals in the same way that treating meat in this manner does. Peppers are rich in carotenoids, folic acid and vitamin C, while hazelnuts are rich in monounsaturated fats.

8 large red peppers (capsicums)
250 g/9 oz spinach leaves, washed
60 g/2 oz hazelnuts
200 g/7 oz low fat cottage cheese
salt and freshly ground black pepper
32 long chives

The best way to prepare the peppers is to place them over a flame and burn their skins off by turning them around so they cook evenly. (Alternatively cut them in half lengthways and place under a hot grill until the skin blackens.) Place them immediately in a plastic bag to cool and then peel off the blackened skins. Remove the seeds and slice the flesh in half lengthways.

Meanwhile, blanch the spinach until soft and drain really well. Place in a bowl. Toast the hazelnuts and crush them in a mortar and pestle. Add the nuts and cheese to the spinach and mix in well. Season to taste.

To assemble the parcels, place a teaspoon of the spinach and cheese filling in each pepper half and roll tightly. Repeat with all 16 pepper halves. Tie each parcel with two long chives to secure them.

Serve four red pepper parcels per person as a light lunch, accompanied by a mixed salad.

Nutritional info per serving
½ dairy portion, 3 vegetable portions, 1 fat portion
Calories 220 kcal/920 kJ; Fat 13 g (monounsaturated 8 g, polyunsaturated 3 g, saturated 2 g); Protein 12 g; Carbohydrate 15 g; Fibre 5 g; Salt 0.6 g

Tofu and Spinach Lasagne

Serves 4
A lasagne with a difference: this combines the goodness of spinach (which contains magnesium, calcium, iron and folic acid) with phytochemical-rich tofu and tomatoes.

8–12 lasagne sheets
1 tbsp olive oil
1 onion, thinly sliced
2 garlic cloves, crushed
200 g/7 oz mushrooms, washed and sliced
400 g/14 oz spinach trimmed, washed and chopped roughly
400 g/14 oz firm tofu
3 tbsp pesto
800 g/1³/₄ lb tomato sauce (see recipe on page 208)

Preheat the oven to 180°C/350°F/gas 4.

Cook the lasagne sheets in boiling water until soft. Drain and separate them, then brush lightly with a little olive oil.

Heat the remaining oil in a frying pan, add the onion, garlic and mushrooms and sauté for 5–6 minutes until the onions are soft. Add the spinach and cook until it is just wilted, about 3–4 minutes.

Place the tofu in a bowl and crumble it with your fingers. Mix in the pesto.

Assemble the lasagne in a shallow square baking dish by placing a third of the tomato sauce on the bottom, then a third of the lasagne sheets, followed by half the vegetable mixture and topping it with a half of the tofu. Repeat the layers in the same order with the final layer being pasta and topped with tomato sauce. Cook for 35–40 minutes. Serve with salad.

Nutritional info per serving
3 vegetable portions, 2 protein portions, 1 ½ fat portions, 2 starchy food portions
Calories 450 kcal/1881 kJ; Fat 15 g (monounsaturated 7 g, polyunsaturated 5 g, saturated 3 g); Protein 25 g; Carbohydrate 50 g; Fibre 7 g; Salt 0.8 g

White Bean and Barley Salad with Yoghurt and Garlic Sauce

Serves 4
Pulses and grains are rich in protein, carbohydrate and minerals and are very easy to use. For this recipe you may use your favourite white beans, for example butter beans or haricots.

$1^1/2$ x 400 g/14 oz cans white beans, rinsed and drained
200 g/7 oz cooked barley (just boiled)
50 g/$1^3/4$ oz sultanas
2 tbsp chopped parsley
2 tbsp chopped thyme
50 g/$1^3/4$ oz walnuts, roughly chopped
6 spring onion, chopped finely
200 g/7 oz baby spinach leaves
salt and freshly ground pepper

YOGHURT AND GARLIC SAUCE
250 ml/8 fl oz thick natural yoghurt
2 garlic cloves, crushed
30 g/1 oz ground walnuts

To make the sauce, place the yoghurt, garlic and walnuts in a food processor and pulse until the mixture is smooth and creamy. Pour into a bowl and chill.

In a large bowl, combine the beans, barley, sultanas, herbs, walnuts and onion and mix well. Season to taste. Add the spinach leaves and toss gently. Serve the salad drizzled with the yoghurt and garlic sauce

Nutritional info per serving
1 vegetable portion, 1 protein portion, 2 starchy food portions, 1½ fat portions
Calories 350 kcal/1463 kJ; Fat 15 g (monounsaturated 4 g, polyunsaturated 10 g, saturated 1 g); Protein 15 g; Carbohydrate 40 g; Fibre 6 g; Salt 0.3 g

Polenta with Kale and Gorgonzola Sauce

Serves 4
Kale is a great brassica that is packed with indole-3-carbinol, folic acid, calcium, magnesium and vitamins C and E.

455 g/1 lb fresh curly kale, washed and cut into small pieces
1 tsp extra virgin olive oil
2 garlic cloves, finely sliced
100 g/3½ oz Gorgonzola or Danish blue cheese, crumbled
1 tbsp fromage frais
200 g/7 oz dry instant polenta
350 ml/12 fl oz water or vegetable stock (made with half
    a stock cube)
salt and freshly ground pepper
2 tbsp chopped fresh chives

Blanch the kale in some boiling water until soft, and drain well. Heat the olive oil in a large saucepan and fry the garlic to just soften. Add the kale and cook for about 3 minutes. Drain and purée the kale and garlic, and keep warm.

Place the Gorgonzola and fromage frais in a small saucepan, mix and heat gently to melt the cheese. Keep warm.

Meanwhile, cook the polenta. Bring the water or stock to boiling point, add the polenta all at once and reduce the heat to low, stirring constantly. The polenta will thicken while cooking. Because we are using instant polenta the cooking process is very quick, about 3–4 minutes. (The polenta should be pourable. If it's too thick, add some more hot water.)

While the polenta is still hot, stir in the spinach purée and serve immediately on individual plates. Drizzle some Gorgonzola sauce over the polenta then sprinkle some chives on top. This dish goes well with a tomato salad or beetroot.

Nutritional info per serving
1 dairy portion, 1 vegetable portion, 2 starchy food portions, 1 fat portion
Calories 310 kcal/1296 kJ; Fat 12 g (monounsaturated 4 g, polyunsaturated 2 g, saturated 6 g); Protein 14 g; Carbohydrate 40 g; Fibre 3 g; Salt 1 g

Broad Beans with Sautéed Tofu

Serves 4
This makes a great filling, low-calorie snack that's super-healthy, too. If you wish to serve it as a meal then use the quantities given below to serve two.

Tofu and broad beans are both packed with phytochemicals; tofu is also rich in calcium while the beans are a good source of folic acid and beta-carotene.

2 tsp extra virgin olive oil
200 g/7 oz firm tofu, cut into cubes
400 g/14 oz fresh or frozen shelled broad beans
2 garlic cloves, crushed
salt and freshly ground pepper
1 tsp sesame oil (optional)

Heat the olive oil in a non-stick frying pan and, when hot, add the tofu cubes and sauté until lightly browned on all sides, about 5 minutes.

Meanwhile, bring a large saucepan of water to the boil. Add the beans and garlic and cook for about 2–3 minutes, until cooked but still firm.

Drain the tofu on kitchen paper and season with salt and pepper. Drain the beans, mix with the sautéed tofu and serve warm, sprinkled with the sesame oil, if using.

Nutritional info per serving
2 protein portions, 1 vegetable portion, 1 fat portion
Calories 110 kcal/460 kJ; Fat 5 g (monounsaturated 2 g, polyunsaturated 2 g, saturated 1 g); Protein 10 g; Carbohydrate 8 g; Fibre 6 g; Salt 0.01 g

Stuffed Courgettes with Almonds and Wild Rice

Serves 4
Courgettes are packed with folic acid, calcium, vitamin C and carotenoids, while almonds are rich in monounsaturated fats, magnesium, calcium and vitamin E.

The stuffing in this recipe also works well with large tomatoes.

8 courgettes (zucchini)
2 tbsp extra virgin olive oil
1 onion, finely chopped
2 garlic cloves, finely chopped
salt and freshly ground pepper
$^{1}/_{2}$ tsp ground allspice
$^{1}/_{2}$ tsp ground cinnamon
180 g/6 oz wild rice
90 g/3 oz chopped almonds
seeds of 2 pomegranates or 50 g/2 oz dried blueberries
4 tbsp chopped parsley

Preheat the oven to 180°C/350°F/gas 4.

First, prepare the courgettes. Halve them lengthways then, using a small sharp knife, carefully hollow them out, removing all the seed pulp from the middle.

To make the stuffing, heat 1 tablespoon of olive oil in a large sauté pan and add the onion, garlic, salt, pepper, allspice and cinnamon. Stir and sauté for about 5 minutes, then add the rice and cook for another 2 minutes, making sure that the rice granules are well coated with the spice mixture. Add about 150 ml/5 fl oz water and cook until the rice is just cooked. Add the almonds, pomegranate seeds and parsley. Cool.

Fill the courgettes with the stuffing and place in an ovenproof dish. Drizzle with the remaining oil and add some water to the base of the dish. Bake, uncovered, for about 30 minutes, basting occasionally with the pan juices. Serve with a crispy green salad.

Nutritional info per serving

2 vegetable portions, 2 starchy food portions, 1 ½ fat portions, ½ fruit portion
Calories 410 kcal/1714 kJ; Fat 19 g (monounsaturated 13 g, polyunsaturated 4 g, saturated 2 g); Protein 12 g; Carbohydrate 45 g; Fibre 4 g ; Salt 0 g

Chicken Poached in Vinegar

Serves 4

This tasty, low fat chicken and carrot recipe is high in zinc, folic acid and beta-carotene.

4 skinless chicken breasts
freshly ground pepper
4 carrots, chopped
2 onions, chopped
3 garlic cloves, sliced
240 ml/8 fl oz white wine vinegar
4 tbsp balsamic vinegar
1 tbsp olive oil spread
1 tbsp tomato purée (paste)
200 ml/7 fl oz chicken stock (made with ¼ of a stock cube)
4 sprigs of thyme
1 small bunch of parsley

Season the chicken with pepper. Place the carrots, onion, garlic, vinegars, olive oil spread, tomato purée, stock and herbs in a deep casserole dish and stir well. Bring to the boil, immediately reduce the heat and simmer for 10 minutes.

Add the chicken, cover and continue to simmer for 20–30 minutes. When cooked, allow the chicken to cool a little before removing from the casserole. Place the casserole back on the heat and simmer until the sauce is reduced by 50 per cent. Return the chicken to the casserole dish, cover with sauce and serve.

Great with boiled or roasted beetroot and a mixed salad.

Nutritional info per serving
4 protein portions, 1 vegetable portion
Calories 220 kcal/924 kJ; Fat 8 g (monounsaturated 4 g, polyunsaturated 2 g, saturated 2 g); Protein 27 g; Carbohydrate 8 g; Fibre 3 g; Salt 0.7 g

Baked Chicken with Olives

Serves 4

The rich tomato sauce in this Mediterranean-style chicken dish is packed with carotenoids.

4 skinless chicken breasts, about 125 g/4½ oz each
80 g/2½ oz pitted green olives, halved
40 g/1¼ oz pitted black olives, halved
4 garlic cloves, halved
1 tbsp extra virgin olive oil
salt and freshly ground pepper
small bunch of parsley, finely chopped
400 g/14 oz cherry tomatoes
juice of 1 lemon

Preheat the oven to 180°C/350°F/gas 4.

Place the chicken breasts in a baking dish, add the olives, garlic, olive oil and seasoning and mix together well. Bake for approximately 25 minutes then add tomatoes and bake for a further 10–12 minutes until the chicken is cooked.

Squeeze over the lemon juice and add the parsley. Serve with boiled or jacket potatoes and a mixed salad.

Nutritional info per serving
4 protein portions, 1 fat portion, 1 vegetable portion
Calories 300 kcal/1254 kJ; Fat 13 g (monounsaturated 7.5 g, polyunsaturated 2.5 g, saturated 3 g); Protein 35 g; Carbohydrate 3 g; Fibre 3 g; Salt 1.7 g

Georgian Meatballs with Pine Nuts and Cranberries

Serves 4

This recipe is influenced by the cuisine of Persia and although it has a long list of ingredients it is simple to prepare and produces great tasting meatballs. Turkey is an excellent low fat meat that is rich in the minerals selenium, zinc and magnesium.

400 g/14 oz minced turkey

1 onion, finely chopped

3 garlic cloves, crushed

50 g/1³/₄ oz dried cranberries

30 g/1 oz pine nuts, roughly chopped and lightly toasted

¼ tsp Hungarian paprika

⅛ tsp cinnamon

⅛ tsp allspice

1 egg white, lightly whipped

small bunch of coriander, finely chopped

small bunch of mint, finely chopped

salt and freshly ground pepper

1 tbsp oil

In a large bowl, combine the minced turkey, onion, garlic, cranberries, pine nuts, paprika, cinnamon and allspice. Mix well then add the egg white and mix again. Finally, add the chopped fresh herbs and seasoning and mix thoroughly. Shape the mixture into small balls (golf ball size).

Heat the oil in a large non-stick frying pan and sauté the meatballs for about 10 minutes until brown on all sides.

Serve at room temperature with bulgur wheat and fresh salad.

Nutritional info per serving
4 protein portions, 1 fat portion
Calories 300 kcal/1254 kJ; Fat 15 g (monounsaturated 5.5 g, polyunsaturated 6 g, saturated 3.5 g); Protein 30 g; Carbohydrate 6 g; Fibre 2 g; Salt 0.2 g

Fennel-Crusted Chicken Breasts with Coriander Gremolata

Serves 4

In this recipe, the crushed fennel and coriander seeds form an aromatic crust when the chicken breasts are cooked.

A great low fat chicken recipe, each serving also provides 20 per cent of the selenium we need each day.

1¹/₂ tbsp fennel seeds
1 tsp coriander seeds
¹/₄ tsp coarsely ground pepper
4 chicken breasts (about 125 g/4¹/₂ oz) each
1 tbsp extra virgin olive oil

GREMOLATA
1 tsp crushed garlic
salt
3 tsp grated lemon zest
juice of 1 lemon
small bunch coriander, finely chopped
2 tsp extra virgin olive oil

Preheat the oven to 180°C/350°F/gas 4.

Roast the fennel and coriander seeds in a heavy frying pan, over moderate heat, until fragrant. Transfer to a spice grinder or mortar and pestle and coarsely grind. Stir in the pepper. Place the mixture on a plate.

Rub some olive oil over the chicken breasts and roll them in the spice mix, pressing gently to ensure the spices adhere.

To make the gremolata, mix the garlic, a little salt, the lemon zest and juice together. Add the coriander and oil and mix well. Set aside.

Place chicken breasts in a roasting tin and bake for 35 minutes. Serve with the gremolata and a crispy green salad and a pasta or potato salad in yoghurt dressing.

Nutritional info per serving
4 protein portions, ¹/₂ fat portion
Calories 250 kcal/1045 kJ; Fat 10 g (monounsaturated 6 g, polyunsaturated 2 g, saturated 2 g); Protein 35 g; Carbohydrate 0 g; Fibre 0 g; Salt 0.2 g

(Wk) Chicken with Grapes and Apricots

Serves 4

The chicken in this delicious fruity recipe has to be marinated, so you need to start preparations the day before. Grapes and grape juice are a great source of the cancer-protective phytochemical resveraterol while sesame seeds are rich in minerals.

1 tbsp runny honey
1 tsp grated fresh root ginger
1 tsp ground cinnamon
1 tsp freshly ground pepper
100 ml/3¹/₂ fl oz grape juice
1.3 kg/2³/₄ lb chicken quarters (chicken breasts can also be used but
    reduce the cooking time)
1 tbsp extra virgin olive oil
1 onion, chopped
2 garlic cloves, crushed
1 cinnamon stick
100 g/3¹/₂ oz seedless grapes, halved
100 g/3¹/₂ oz fresh apricots, pitted
2 tbsp sesame seeds, toasted

In a large bowl combine the honey, ginger, cinnamon, pepper and grape juice, stirring together. Rub the mixture over the chicken and let it marinate in the refrigerator overnight, covered.

Heat the olive oil in a large sauté pan, add the onion and garlic and sauté until the onion is just golden in colour. Drain the chicken, reserving the marinade, and add the chicken pieces to the pan. Brown all the pieces evenly. Now add the chicken marinade, 300 ml/10 fl oz of water and the cinnamon stick, and simmer for 20–30 minutes. By this point the liquid should have reduced by about half, and the chicken pieces should be cooked.

Finally add the grapes and apricot halves and simmer for a further 5–8 minutes. Serve immediately, sprinkled with the sesame seeds, and accompanied by boiled brown rice and salad.

Nutritional info per serving
4 protein portions, 1 fruit portion, 1 fat portion
Calories 330 kcal/1379 kJ; Fat 13 g (monounsaturated 7 g, polyunsaturated 4 g,
saturated 2 g); Protein 40 g; Carbohydrate 15 g; Fibre 2 g; Salt 0.2 g

(Fm) Chicken- and Tabbouleh-stuffed Pittas with Yoghurt Dressing

Serves 4

Wholegrain bulgur wheat and wholemeal pitta makes this a
satisfying wholesome meal that is packed with fibre and
phytochemicals. Each serving provides 40 per cent of the
magnesium and 20 per cent of the selenium we require each day.

4 skinless chicken breasts
3 tbsp harissa (north African chilli paste)
freshly ground pepper
125 g/4½ oz bulgur wheat
2 garlic cloves, crushed
1 small red onion
5 tbsp fresh chopped coriander
4 pitta breads

YOGHURT DRESSING
100 ml/3½ fl oz low fat natural yoghurt
4 tbsp tahini (sesame seed paste)
juice of 1 lemon
salt and freshly ground pepper

Rub the chicken breast with the harissa, season with pepper and
set aside to marinate for at least 4 hours.

To make the tabbouleh, wash the bulgur wheat, place in a
saucepan and boil for about 20 minutes. Drain and season. Mix
in the garlic, onion and coriander. Set aside until ready to use.

Cook the chicken in a 180°C/350°F/gas 4 oven for about
20 minutes, turning frequently, until cooked. Cut into
1 cm/½ in slices.

To prepare the yoghurt dressing, mix together the yoghurt, tahini and lemon juice. Season with salt and pepper and mix well.

To assemble, place the pittas on the hot grill for a minute or so on each side and cut the breads in half into small pockets. Place some chicken, tabbouleh and dressing in each pitta. Serve with a green salad.

Nutritional info per serving

3 starchy food portions, 4 protein portions, 1/2 fat portion

Calories 540 kcal/2257 kJ; Fat 12 g (monounsaturated 5 g, polyunsaturated 4 g, saturated fat 3 g); Protein 40 g; Carbohydrate 70 g; Fibre 6 g; Salt 1 g

(Fm) Tarragon Roast Chicken with Sweet Potato and Pumpkin Crumble

Serves 4

Roast chicken and tarragon is a classic combination. As a general rule it is always best to use fresh herbs but in the case of tarragon, and tarragon only, dried is also fine. The accompanying dish is a delicious combination of orange-fleshed sweet potatoes and pumpkin. This is a good way of getting children to eat pumpkin, which is rich in cancer-protective beta-carotene.

4 large chicken breasts with bone in, skin removed
1 tbsp extra virgin olive oil
juice of 1 lemon
3 tbsp tarragon leaves
4 tbsp red grape juice
salt and freshly ground pepper

SWEET POTATO AND PUMPKIN CRUMBLE
3 large orange-fleshed sweet potatoes, peeled and diced
100 g/3½ oz pumpkin, peeled and diced
20 g/¾ oz olive oil spread
1 tbsp maple syrup
¼ tsp grated nutmeg

salt and freshly ground pepper
100 g/3¹/₂ oz fresh breadcrumbs, preferably wholemeal
3 tbsp chopped chives

Preheat the oven to 180°C/350°F/gas 4.

Place the skinned chicken in a large roasting tin. Rub the olive oil into the chicken, pour the lemon juice all over and sprinkle with two-thirds of the tarragon, salt and pepper. Add the grape juice, cover with foil and cook in the oven for 20 minutes. Remove the foil, sprinkle the remainder of the tarragon over the chicken breasts and continue cooking for another 25 minutes.

Meanwhile, make the crumble. Cook the potatoes and squash in boiling salted water until soft. Drain and add the olive oil spread, maple syrup, nutmeg, salt and pepper. Purée in a food processor and spoon into a medium baking dish.

Toast the breadcrumbs in a dry sauté pan until only just brown then sprinkle over the top of the crumble. Bake in the pre-heated oven for 20–30 minutes until golden brown.

Nutritional info per serving
4 protein portions, 1 starchy food portion, 1 fat portion
Calories 400 kcal/1672 kJ; Fat 13 g (monounsaturated 7.5 g, polyunsaturated 2.5 g, saturated 3 g); Protein 40 g; Carbohydrate 35 g; Fibre 4 g; Salt 0.3 g

FISH

Steamed Halibut, wrapped in Pak Choi with Broad Bean, Feta and Spinach Mash

Serves 4

Steamed fish keeps its taste and nutritional value. This recipe combines the goodness of fish (which is rich in magnesium and vitamin E) with that of pak choi (rich in the cancer-protective phytochemical indole-3-carbinol) and spinach and beans (which contain folic acid, calcium, magnesium and carotenoids). That's a lot of goodness in one meal.

4 x 180 g/6¹/₂ oz halibut pieces, skin removed
freshly ground pepper
8 large pak choi (bok choy) leaves, blanched
   and trimmed

MASH
400 g/14 oz shelled broad beans (use frozen beans if
   fresh are unavailable)
100 g/3¹/₂ oz low fat sheep's feta cheese
200 g/7 oz baby spinach leaves
4 tsp extra virgin olive oil
small bunch of fresh mint

Season the halibut with pepper. Place two pak choi leaves end to end, place a piece of halibut in the centre and wrap the leaves around the fish, slightly exposing the ends of the fillet. Repeat for each piece of fish. Place in a steamer and steam for 6 minutes (it is possible to steam this dish in a colander over a pan of boiling water if you do not have a steamer).

   Meanwhile, make the broad bean mash. Cook the beans in boiling water for about 8–10 minutes until soft, then place in a food processor together with the feta cheese and the baby spinach; add the oil and mint and pulse until relatively smooth.

Serve the mash warm and accompanied by the steamed halibut, still wrapped in the pak choi.

Nutritional info per serving
4 protein food portions, 1 dairy portion, 1 fat portion, 2 vegetable portions
Calories 370 kcal/1547 kJ; Fat 15 g (monounsaturated 7 g, polyunsaturated 3 g, saturated 5 g); Protein 50 g; Carbohydrate 10 g; Fibre 8 g; Salt 1.2 g

Sesame-crusted Salmon with Asian Greens and Ginger Salsa

Serves 4

This delicious salmon recipe is packed with lots of good things. Each portion provides 70 per cent of the vitamin D, half of the selenium, 30 per cent of the folic acid, 25 per cent of the magnesium and 20 per cent of the calcium we need each day.

4 x 125 g/4½ oz salmon fillets
2 egg whites, lightly beaten
2 tbsp white sesame seeds
1 tbsp extra virgin olive oil
400 g/14 oz Chinese cabbage, washed and sliced thinly
1 bunch spring onions, trimmed and finely sliced
1 tbsp soy sauce

GINGER SALSA
3 cm/1¼ in piece fresh ginger, finely grated
1 red chilli, deseeded and finely sliced
handful of coriander leaves, chopped
juice of 1 lime
1 tsp sesame oil

Dip the salmon fillets in egg white then roll them in the sesame seeds, pressing lightly to coat them evenly on all sides.

Heat a heavy non-stick pan, add the salmon and cook for 3 minutes on each side. Keep warm.

Meanwhile, heat the oil in a wok, add the Chinese cabbage and spring onions and stir-fry for 2–3 minutes. Add the soy sauce.

To make the ginger salsa, place all the salsa ingredients in a mixing bowl and mix well to combine.

Serve the sesame-crusted salmon on top of the greens, garnished with the fresh ginger salsa. Accompany with boiled brown rice and an additional portion of steamed vegetables.

Nutritional info per serving
4 protein portions, 1 vegetable portion
Calories 320 kcal/1338 kJ; Fat 18 g (monounsaturated 9 g, polyunsaturated 6 g, saturated 3 g); Protein 30 g; Carbohydrate 4 g; Fibre 2 g; Salt 1.5 g

Roasted Fillet of Lemon Sole on Watercress and Sweet Potato Cake

Serves 4

Watercress is great combined with fish and it's packed with cancer-protective indole-3-carbinol, calcium, magnesium, vitamin C and beta-carotene. The sweet potatoes further boost the beta-carotene content of this recipe.

280 g/10 oz watercress, washed (or use a mixture of watercress and spinach)
400 g/14 oz sweet potatoes, cubed
salt and freshly ground pepper
80 g/2½ oz plain flour
1 egg, beaten
3 tbsp sesame seeds
2 tbsp extra virgin olive oil

4 x 150 g/5½ oz fillets lemon sole
10 g olive oil spread, melted
large handful of basil leaves for garnish

Preheat the oven to 180°C/350°F/gas 4.

Begin by making the potato cakes. Boil the sweet potatoes until cooked, about 10 minutes, and then mash. Place the watercress in a small saucepan with a little water and heat, stirring often, until wilted. Drain well and chop the leaves finely or pulse in a food processor. Place the mashed potato and watercress in a bowl and mix together. Season well. Divide the mixture into four balls; shape them into cakes that are large enough to sit the fish fillets on top and place in the refrigerator to firm up until ready to cook.

Meanwhile, place the lemon sole fillets in a shallow ovenproof dish and brush with the melted olive oil spread. Season and keep chilled until ready to cook.

Coat the potato cakes with flour, dusting off any excess, then dip into the egg, coating evenly. Now coat the cakes well with sesame seeds. Heat the oil in a frying pan, add the potato cakes, and cook on a medium heat for about 4 minutes each side. Transfer them to a baking sheet and cook in the oven for another 12 minutes.

Place the dish containing the fillets in the hot oven for about 8–10 minutes until they are just cooked and flake easily.

To serve, place a potato cake in the centre of each plate and top with a lemon sole fillet. Garnish with basil leaves and serve with a green or mixed salad.

Nutritional info per serving
3 protein food portions, 1 vegetable portion, 1 starchy food portion, 1 fat portion
Calories 430 kcal/1797 kJ; Fat 17 g (monounsaturated 9 g, polyunsaturated 5 g, saturated 3 g); Protein 35 g; Carbohydrate 35 g; Fibre 5 g; Salt 0.6 g

(Fm) Tuna and Avocado Burgers with Bean Curd Aioli

Serves 4
This is a healthy alternative to beef burgers. The avocado gives the burgers a delicate, soft texture, and the bean curd aioli is a great alternative to the usual fattening dressings. Tuna, especially fresh tuna, is an excellent source of the omega-3 fish oils.

480 g/17 oz fresh tuna or canned if fresh is unavailable
1 large shallot, finely chopped
2 garlic cloves, finely chopped
1 tsp finely grated ginger
1 small green chilli, finely chopped
1 avocado, peeled and diced
2 tbsp light soy sauce
salt and freshly ground pepper
1 tbsp extra virgin olive oil

BEAN CURD AIOLI
180 g/6½ oz fresh silken tofu
juice of 1 lemon
2 tbsp extra virgin olive oil
3 garlic cloves, crushed
salt and freshly ground pepper

Finely chop the tuna, but do not mince it, as this will spoil the chunky, homemade texture of the burgers. Place the tuna in a bowl and add the shallot, garlic, ginger, chilli, avocado and soy sauce. Season with salt and pepper and, using your hands, mix lightly, making sure that you do not squash the diced avocado too much. Shape into four burgers and chill them until you are ready to cook.

To make the bean curd aioli, place the tofu in a food processor, add the seasoning and lemon juice and, with the machine running, slowly add the olive oil until the mixture is smooth. Finally add the garlic and check seasoning.

Brush the burgers with a little olive oil, place under a preheated grill and cook for 3–4 minutes on each side. Serve with some bean curd aioli.

Nutritional info per serving
4 protein food portions, 2 fat portions
Calories 375 kcal/1567 kJ; Fat 18 g (monounsaturated 12 g, polyunsaturated 3 g, saturated fat 3 g); Protein 35 g; Carbohydrate 5 g; Fibre 2 g; Salt 0.2 g

(Wk) Citrus Salmon served with Bulgur Pilaf

Serves 4

Try to use wild salmon for this dish as it is richer in omega-3 fats than the farmed variety. This recipe is packed with phytochemicals from the citrus fruit and each portion also contains an impressive 60 per cent of the omega-3 fats and 70 per cent of the vitamin D we need each day.

500 g/1 lb 2 oz wild salmon fillet, skin and pin
   bones removed

CITRUS MARINADE
finely grated zest and juice of ¹/₂ lemon, ¹/₂ orange, ¹/₂ lime
   and ¹/₄ grapefruit
¹/₂ tbsp sugar
¹/₄ tbsp freshly ground white pepper

BULGUR PILAF
1 shallot, finely chopped
2 garlic cloves, crushed
1 tbsp extra virgin olive oil
200 g/7 oz bulgur wheat
300 ml/10 fl oz vegetable stock (made with ¹/₄ of a stock cube)
40 g/1¹/₄ oz semi-dry mango, chopped into small pieces
30 g/1 oz currants
30 g/1 oz toasted pine nuts
small bunch of coriander, finely chopped

Combine the marinade ingredients in a bowl.

Cut out a piece of foil large enough to envelope the fish fillet. Place the fish on the foil and coat with the zesty marinade. Bring the sides of the foil together over the top of the fish and roll the foil down to form a packet. Place the fish in the refrigerator to marinate for about 2 hours.

Remove the fish from the foil and rinse off the marinade. Dry the fillet well and cut into four portions. Place the fillets in a steamer and cook for about 6–8 minutes. To test if the salmon is cooked, remove a piece and bend it slightly, it should begin to flake. When cooked, remove the salmon and keep warm.

Meanwhile, prepare the pilaf. Sauté the shallots and garlic in the oil, over medium heat, until the shallots are translucent in colour. Add the bulgur and stir to coat the grains with the olive oil. Slowly add the stock and reduce the heat to low, stirring until all the liquid is absorbed, about 8 minutes. Add the mango and currants, mix well and top with the pine nuts. Keep warm until ready to use.

To serve, place some bulgur pilaf onto the centre of a dinner plate and top with a piece of citrus salmon. Sprinkle with fresh coriander. Serve with steamed vegetables or a salad.

Nutritional info per serving
4 protein portions, 2 starchy food portions, 1 fat portion
Calories 500 kcal/2090 kJ; Fat 20 g (monounsaturated 8 g, polyunsaturated 9 g, saturated 3 g); Protein 30 g; Carbohydrate 50 g; Fibre 2 g; Salt 0.4 g

(Fm) Monkfish Plaki

Serves 4
Plaki is a Greek and Bulgarian method of baking fish. The fish is cooked with lots of wonderful vegetables, making the dish simple as well as delicious. As well as monkfish, you can prepare plaki with other kinds of fish, such as cod or sea bass.

Tomatoes, spinach and olives are packed with phytochemicals and vitamins, while walnuts are a great source of omega-3 fats. Each serving provides all of the vitamin E requirement for a day, as well as significant amounts of folic acid, vitamin C, beta-carotene and lycopene.

600 g/1 lb 5 oz monkfish fillet
3 tbsp extra virgin olive oil
2 onions, chopped

3 garlic cloves, chopped
300 g/10^1/$_2$ oz chopped tomatoes
100 ml/3^1/$_2$ fl oz red grape juice
100 g/3^1/$_2$ oz spinach, washed and chopped
100 g/3^1/$_2$ oz green olives
5 tbsp chopped parsley
5 tbsp chopped basil
60 g/2 oz walnuts, coarsely chopped
200 g/7 oz brown rice

Preheat the oven to 180°C/350°F/gas 4.

Rinse the fish, cut it into chunks and set aside.

Place the oil in a large sauté pan, add the onions and garlic and fry gently until the onions are soft and golden. Make sure that they don't brown too much. Add the tomatoes, grape juice and 100 ml/3½ fl oz water, bring to boil and simmer for 10 minutes (the cooking liquid should be reduced by this point).

Stir in the spinach and olives. Now place the monkfish pieces on the top. Season and simmer gently for about 8 minutes. Add the walnuts and half the herbs and transfer everything to a deep heavy casserole. Cover with foil and cook in the oven for 15 minutes.

Meanwhile, boil the brown rice. When the fish is ready, sprinkle with the remaining herbs and serve accompanied by the rice and a green salad or steamed vegetables.

Nutritional info per serving (with rice)
3 protein portions, 2 starchy food portions, 1 fat portion
Calories 500 kcal/2090 kJ; Fat 17 g (monounsaturated 7 g, polyunsaturated 8 g, saturated 2 g); Protein 30 g; Carbohydrate 50 g; Fibre 5 g; Salt 0.3 g

(Fm) Salmon Teriyaki with Cucumber Salsa

Serves 4

The salmon in this recipe needs to marinate for at least 3 hours before cooking. This helps ensure that harmful chemicals are not produced when the fish is grilled.

This recipe has a wide range of cancer fighting nutrients: salmon is a great source of omega-3 fats, vitamins D and E, and selenium; the herbs and vegetables contain phytochemicals. Each portion provides 50 per cent of the omega-3 fat, 40 per cent of the selenium, 70 per cent of the vitamin D, and three-quarters of the vitamin E recommended each day.

4 salmon steaks, weighing about 125 g/4^{1}/$_2$ oz each

TERIYAKI MARINADE
4 tbsp dry sherry (or water mixed with a few drops of
    Angostura bitters)
3 tbsp soy sauce
2 tbsp brown sugar
3 garlic cloves, crushed
2 tbsp lemon juice
freshly ground pepper

SALSA
3 tbsp extra virgin olive oil
2 garlic cloves, crushed
100 g/3^{1}/$_2$ oz broad beans
2 tbsp fresh mint, chopped
2 tbsp fresh dill, chopped
1 cucumber, peeled and grated
1^{1}/$_2$ tsp rice vinegar
freshly ground pepper

Mix all the marinade ingredients in a shallow dish, adding pepper to taste. Place the fish steaks in the marinade, making sure that they are covered. Cover with cling film and place in the refrigerator to marinate for at least 3 hours (but no longer than 8 hours).

To make the salsa, cook the broad beans in water until soft, then drain and purée in a food processor with the olive oil, garlic and herbs until smooth. Add the cucumber and rice vinegar and season to taste.

Remove the fish from the marinade and cook under a preheated grill about 6–8 minutes each side. Keep brushing the fish with the marinade while it is cooking.

Serve the fish accompanied by the cucumber salsa.

Nutritional info per serving
4 protein portions, 1 fat portion
Calories 430 kcal/1797 kJ; Fat 27 g (monounsaturated 14 g, polyunsaturated 8 g, saturated 5 g); Protein 25 g; Carbohydrate 15 g; Fibre 2 g; Salt 1 g

(Wk) Pan-fried Fish with Beetroot Purée and Roast Sweet Potatoes

Serves 4

Beetroot are rich in phytochemicals and a great source of folic acid. This recipe combines them with the goodness of fish (which contains magnesium, selenium and vitamin E) and sweet potatoes (which are rich in beta-carotene).

The type of beetroot specified in this recipe has a lovely flavour but you can use ordinary beetroot if you wish.

400 g/14 oz orange-fleshed sweet potatoes, peeled and sliced into 1 cm/¹/₂ in thick slices
4 x 150 g/5¹/₂ oz fillets haddock or cod
plain flour
2 tbsp extra virgin olive oil

BEETROOT PURÉE

2 shallots, finely chopped

1 tbsp fresh thyme

1 tbsp extra virgin olive oil

1 rasher smoked bacon (optional)

4 large Burpees golden beetroots, washed, peeled and chopped into small
  pieces (ordinary beetroot can be substituted)

150 ml/5 fl oz natural yoghurt

freshly ground pepper

First prepare the sweet potatoes. Boil them for about 3 minutes
until only semi-soft. Drain them well, brush with oil and roast
them in a hot oven for 20–25 minutes, or until browned.

Meanwhile, prepare the beetroot purée. Sweat the shallot and
thyme in the olive oil, then add the bacon and continue cooking.
Add the beetroot pieces and cook until they are soft, about 20
minutes. Finally add the yoghurt and simmer for few more
minutes (do not boil). Season with pepper, liquidize and pass
through a sieve. Keep warm.

Remove the skin from the fish. Coat the fish with plain flour.
Heat the olive oil in a heavy frying pan and, when hot enough,
pan-fry the fish for about 3 minutes on each side.

To serve, spoon some beetroot purée onto the middle of each
serving plate, place a fillet of pan-fried fish on the top and serve
the roast sweet potatoes alongside. Accompany with two portions
of steamed green vegetables.

Nutritional info per serving
4 protein portions, 1 starchy food portion, 1 vegetable portion, ½ fat portion
Calories 320 kcal/1338 kJ; Fat 8 g (monounsaturated 4 g, polyunsaturated 2 g,
saturated 2 g); Protein 35 g; Carbohydrate 30 g; Fibre 4 g; Salt 0.7 g

MEAT

(Fm) Cottage Pie with Cauliflower Topping

Serves 4

This is an unusual version of the classic cottage pie recipe. Instead of the traditional potato topping this version uses a cauliflower purée. In order to minimize the amount of saturated fat, use the leanest minced beef available.

Cauliflower is a great source of the anti-cancer chemical indole-3-carbinol, and carotenoids. This dish is also a good source of calcium, zinc, iron and selenium.

400 g/14 oz lean minced beef
1 large onion, finely chopped
100 g/3^1/$_2$ oz cooked lentils
3 carrots, diced
3 tsp Worcestershire sauce
250 ml/8 fl oz stock
1 large cauliflower, cut into small florets
20 g/^{3}/$_4$ oz olive oil spread
4 tbsp milk
salt and freshly ground pepper
small bunch of parsley, finely chopped
100 g/3^1/$_2$ oz grated low fat Cheddar

Place the minced beef and onion in a large frying pan and cook over medium heat until the meat is no longer pink, breaking it up with a fork. Drain any fat off and add the lentils, carrots, Worcestershire sauce and stock. Simmer for about 30 minutes then spoon into a shallow baking dish.

While the meat is cooking, prepare the cauliflower topping. Place the florets in a saucepan with some water and cook on medium heat until they are soft. Drain and add the olive oil spread and milk. Season with salt and pepper, and mash as you would potatoes. Stir in the parsley. Don't worry if the cauliflower mash is not as smooth as a potato mash. This is due to the different texture of cauliflower.

Spoon the mashed cauliflower on top of the meat and sprinkle with the cheese. Bake for 40 minutes at 190°C/375°F/gas 5 until golden brown. Serve hot.

Nutritional info per serving
4 protein portions, 1 dairy portion, 1 fat portion
Calories 350 kcal/1463 kJ; Fat 17 g (monounsaturated 7 g, polyunsaturated 3 g,
saturated 7 g); Protein 35 g; Carbohydrate 14 g; Fibre 3 g; Salt 1 g

(Wk) Braised Fillet of Lamb with Prunes and Apricots

Serves 4

Lamb is complemented beautifully by the subtle sweetness of the prunes in this recipe.

Each serving provides 40 per cent of our daily iron and zinc requirements.

200 ml/7 fl oz very strong black or Chinese tea
100 g/3^{1}/$_{2}$ oz prunes
80 g/2^{1}/$_{2}$ oz dried apricots, halved
1 tbsp olive oil
1 large onion, finely chopped
400 g/14 oz lamb fillet (from the leg), cubed
2 tbsp plain flour
salt and freshly ground pepper
200 ml/7 fl oz lamb stock (made from the lamb bones if possible
    or ^{1}/$_{3}$rd of a stock cube)
5 tbsp white wine vinegar
2 bay leaves
^{1}/$_{2}$ tsp ground cinnamon
pinch of ground cloves

Bring the tea to a boil and pour over the prunes and apricots. Leave to stand for an hour. Remove the fruit and set aside.

Heat the oil in a casserole dish, add the onion and sauté until lightly coloured. Meanwhile, dust the meat with flour, season and add to the casserole. Cook, stirring frequently, until the meat is browned. Add the stock and simmer until the sauce has slightly thickened, about 20–30 minutes.

Add the vinegar, bay leaves, cinnamon, cloves and fruit. Bring to a boil and simmer for about 20 minutes until the meat is tender. Serve hot, with brown rice, couscous or bulgur wheat.

Nutritional info per serving
4 protein portions, 1 fruit portion, ½ fat portion
Calories 340 kcal/1421 kJ; Fat 12 g (monounsaturated 5 g, polyunsaturated 1 g, saturated 6 g); Protein 25 g; Carbohydrate 30 g; Fibre 5 g; Salt 0.5 g

(Wk) Pork- and Quince-stuffed Chard Leaves

Serves 4

Some of the ingredients in this recipe are not available all year round but that's one of the joys of fresh seasonal produce. However, you can enjoy variations on it at any time by using more common ingredients: when chard leaves are unavailable, use vine leaves or large spinach leaves and when quince is out of season use apple or pear.

This tasty low fat recipe provides good nutrition, too. The pork provides iron and selenium whilst chard contains magnesium, folic acid, vitamin C and carotenoids.

20 Swiss chard leaves, washed
1 large quince
4 tbsp lemon juice
1 tbsp liquid honey

FILLING
400 g/14 oz minced pork
small bunch of parsley, finely chopped
125 g/4^1/2 oz long-grain rice, cooked
1 small onion, finely chopped
salt and freshly ground pepper

Preheat the oven to 160°C/325°F/gas 3.

Trim the Swiss chard, place it in a large saucepan filled with hot water and blanch for 1–2 minutes.

To make the filling, mix together the pork, parsley, rice and onion and season well.

Spread each Swiss chard leaf on your work surface and place a spoonful of the meat mixture in the middle. Fold over the top and roll up, tucking in both sides like a small parcel. Use wooden toothpicks to secure the parcels. Place the stuffed chard leaves in a single layer, seam down, in a wide but deep baking dish.

Peel, core and cut the quince into 1 cm/$\frac{1}{2}$ in thick slices. Place on top of the chard parcels. Mix the lemon juice and honey with 2 tablespoons of water and drizzle over the parcels. Cover the dish well with foil, and cook in the oven for about one hour. Serve immediately.

Nutritional info per serving
4 protein portions, 2 vegetable portions, 1 starchy food portion
Calories 350 kcal/1463 kJ; Fat 10 g (monounsaturated 4 g, polyunsaturated 2 g, saturated 4 g); Protein 25 g; Carbohydrate 40 g; Fibre 2 g; Salt 1 g

DESSERTS

Apricot, Almond and Apple Salad

Serves 4

This simple fruit salad is a lovely concoction, with a great combination of textures. It's also packed with beta-carotene.

100 g/3½ oz dried apricots
4 small crisp apples
50 g/1¾ oz flaked almonds, toasted

Place the apricots in a shallow dish, pour over just enough water to cover them and soak overnight.

When you are ready to serve the salad, core the apples and cut into thin slices. Mix the apple slices with the apricots and top with toasted flaked almonds. Serve immediately.

Nutritional info per serving
2 fruit portions, 1 fat portion
Calories 200 kcal/836 kJ; Fat 11 g (monounsaturated 7 g, polyunsaturated 3 g, saturated 1 g); Protein 6 g; Carbohydrate 20 g; Fibre 5 g; Salt 0.5 g

Balsamic Roasted Pears with Feta and Honey

Serves 4

The savoury cheese flavours work beautifully with the sweet intonations of the pears and the honey. Each serving provides 20 per cent of your daily calcium requirement.

4 large, slightly under-ripe pears
2 tbsp olive oil spread
3 tbsp balsamic vinegar
4 x 30 g (1 oz) slices feta cheese
3 tbsp pure honey

Preheat the oven to 200°C/400°F/gas 6.

Halve and core the pears but do not peel.

Melt the olive oil spread in a non-stick ovenproof, heavy pan and when just beginning to bubble, add the pears, cut sides down. Sauté for 2 minutes then place in hot oven to cook for 15 minutes. Add vinegar and cook for further 5 minutes. Remove the dish from the oven, drizzle the pears with honey and allow to rest for a few minutes.

Serve warm, drizzled with the cooking juices and accompanied with the slices of feta cheese.

Nutritional info per serving
1 fruit portion, 1 dairy portion, 1 fat portion
Calories 230 kcal/966 kJ; Fat 10 g (monounsaturated 3.5 g, polyunsaturated 1 g, saturated 5.5 g); Protein 6 g; Carbohydrate 32 g; Fibre 4 g; Salt 1.2 g

Rhubarb and Elderflower Jelly

Serves 4
Rhubarb is packed with fibre and is a great source of vitamin C and calcium: each serving provides 20 per cent of the calcium and about a quarter of the vitamin C you need each day.

The jelly, once cooked, looks too good to eat! Blood oranges are used to intensify the bright colours but if these are unavailable ordinary oranges will suffice.

455 g/1lb fresh English rhubarb
50 g/1³/₄ oz caster sugar
5 tbsp elderflower cordial
11 g sachet of gelatine granules
juice of 2 small blood oranges

Chop the rhubarb into 2 cm/3/4 in pieces and place in a medium saucepan. Add the sugar, elderflower cordial and about 150 ml/5 fl oz of water. Simmer gently on a very low heat until the rhubarb is very soft, about 5 minutes.

Place the hot rhubarb mixture in a food processor and pulse to a smooth purée. Place a sieve over the top of a bowl and strain the liquid out of the rhubarb mixture, pressing with the back of a spoon. Reserve the fruit pulp as well as the juice.

Dissolve half the gelatine in a little hot water, add it to the hot rhubarb juice and mix to dissolve. Pour the liquid into a shallow glass dish and leave to cool. Place in the refrigerator to set.

Meanwhile, place the fruit pulp in a small saucepan, add the orange juice and slowly heat up. Repeat the same procedure with the remaining gelatine as above and once ready add to the hot purée. Keep aside to cool.

Once the rhubarb jelly in the refrigerator has set, pour over the rhubarb purée and spread evenly. Cover and leave to set. The final result is a serving of a beautifully transparent layer of pink jelly, topped with an intensely coloured and textured jelly of fruit.

Nutritional info per serving
1 fruit serving
Calories 100 kcal/418 kJ; Fat 0; Protein 2 g; Carbohydrate 25 g; Fibre 3 g; Salt 0.03 g

Cardamom and Pomegranate Roasted Figs with Pomegranate Sabayon

Serves 4

Figs, pomegranates and cardamom go beautifully together as they are all reminiscent of warm Mediterranean climates, exotic settings and sweet spices. Nectarines also work well in this recipe.

Pomegranates and figs are packed with cancer-protective phytochemicals and beta-carotene, so make the most of their brief seasons. Each serving provides a quarter of your daily beta-carotene requirement.

8 large figs
juice of 2 pomegranates
1¹/₂ tbsp molasses
seeds of 8 cardamom pods, crushed

SABAYON
3 egg yolks
1 tbsp caster sugar
1 tbsp white wine
juice of 1/2 pomegranate

Preheat the oven to 180°C/350°F/gas 4.

Cut a cross in each of the figs, about halfway down, and place them in a shallow baking dish. Mix together the pomegranate juice, molasses and crushed cardamom. Pour this over the figs, and cook in the oven for 15 minutes, basting every now and again with the juices.

Meanwhile, place the ingredients for the sabayon in a heatproof bowl set over simmering water. Cook, whisking constantly, until the mixture has thickened.

Place two figs on each plate and pour over the sabayon.

Nutritional info per serving
1 fruit portion, 1 fat portion
Calories 180 kcal/752 kJ; Fat 8 g (monounsaturated 3 g, polyunsaturated 3 g, saturated 2 g); Protein 4 g; Carbohydrate 25 g; Fibre 2 g; Salt 0.05 g

Lemon and Watermelon Granita

Serves 4
Watermelons are rich in lycopene, while lemon rind is packed with the phytochemical limonene.

2 lemons
455 g/1 lb watermelon, rind and seeds removed
    and flesh chopped
1 1/2 tbsp caster sugar

Grate the rind off the two lemons and extract the juice. Place the juice and grated rind in a blender along with the chopped watermelon, sugar and 80 ml/3 fl oz water. Blend for 1 minute.

Pour the mixture into a shallow dish and freeze. When frozen, break into pieces, place in the blender and blend for 1 minute. Return to the freezer and fork through prior to serving.

If you wish, serve the granita in pieces of the watermelon shell.

Nutritional info per serving
1 fruit portion
Calories 70 kcal/293 kJ; Fat 0g; Protein 1 g; Carbohydrate 15 g; Fibre 0.2 g; Salt 0 g

Ginger Oranges

Serves 2

This recipe is a great way to enjoy vitamin C-rich oranges and the lovely flavour of ginger, which contains the anti-cancer phytochemical gingerol. Each serving provides 30 per cent of the vitamin C you need each day.

1 large orange
1 piece stem ginger in syrup
2 tbsp low fat natural yoghurt

Preheat the grill to medium.

Cut the orange in half and remove any large seeds. To make the halves easier to eat, loosen each section with a serrated knife by cutting between the membranes and around the pith.

Chop the ginger into small dice and scatter over the orange halves. Drizzle about 2 teaspoons of the ginger syrup over each half and place them on a baking tray. Grill for about 5 minutes, or until the tops begin to turn golden.

Eat straight away with a dollop of low fat yoghurt on top.

Nutritional info per serving
1 fruit portion
Calories 70 kcal/293 kJ; Fat 0.5 g (monounsaturated 0.2 g, polyunsaturated 0 g, saturated 0.3 g); Protein 2 g; Carbohydrate 15 g; Fibre 2 g; Salt 0.8 g

Tofu with Ginger and Lime

Serves 4

Tofu is the basis for this filling, tasty dessert. The soya, ginger and lime in this recipe make it a great source of phytochemicals. It is also a good source of calcium; each serving provides 40 per cent of your daily requirement.

5 tbsp soft brown sugar
4 slices fresh root ginger, finely chopped, plus a little extra finely grated or shaved, to garnish
200 g/7 oz fresh silken tofu, drained
6 wedges lime or lemon

Put the sugar and 500 ml/18 fl oz of water in a small saucepan. Place over a low heat and stir until the sugar dissolves. Now add the finely chopped ginger, raise the heat and bring the syrup to a boil. Simmer steadily for 10–15 minutes, stirring occasionally, until the syrup has become a caramel sauce thick enough to lightly coat the back of a spoon (you should have about 5 tablespoons of sauce).

Meanwhile, cut the tofu into neat cubes and place on a serving dish. Sprinkle with a little finely grated ginger. When the caramel sauce is ready, remove from the heat and allow to cool slightly. Pour the sauce through a sieve over the tofu. Serve with the wedges of lime to squeeze over the tofu just before eating.

Nutritional info per serving
1 protein portion
Calories 140 kcal/585 kJ; Fat 2 g (monounsaturated 0.5 g, polyunsaturated 1 g, saturated 0.5 g); Protein 5 g; Carbohydrate 20 g; Fibre 0 g; Salt 0.01 g

Mango Sorbet

Serves 4

Mangoes are a great source of vitamin C and, like other yellow and orange coloured fruits, are packed with cancer-protective carotenoids. Each serving provides a quarter of the vitamin C and all of the beta-carotene recommended each day.

3 mangoes, peeled, stoned and chopped
juice of 1 lime
50 g/1³/₄ oz sugar
2 egg whites

Place the chopped mango, lime juice, sugar and water in a food processor, and process to form a smooth mango purée.

Transfer the mango mixture to a saucepan. Bring to a boil then set aside to cool.

Whisk the egg whites until just frothy. Fold the whisked egg whites into the cooled mango purée.

Freeze the mango mixture in an ice cream maker, following the manufacturer's instructions, or transfer the mixture to a shallow freezer-proof container and freeze until set.

Nutritional info per serving
1 fruit portion
125 kcal/418 kJ; Fat 0.2 g (monounsaturated 0 g, polyunsaturated 0.1 g, saturated 0.1 g); Protein 2.3 g; Carbohydrate 30 g; Fibre 3 g; Salt 0 g

Angel's Food Cake

Serves 10

This is a healthy, low-calorie version of the more devilish chocolate food cake was one of my mum's specialities. The plain chocolate and cocoa in this recipe are rich in flavenols.

300 g/10^1/$_2$ oz sweet potatoes
90 g/3 oz wholemeal flour
90 g/3 oz plain flour
70 g/2^1/$_2$ oz cocoa powder
1 tsp baking powder
50 g/1^3/$_4$ oz 70%-cocoa chocolate, grated
75 g/2^1/$_2$ oz olive oil spread
75 g/2^1/$_2$ oz brown sugar
1 tsp vanilla essence
3 eggs

Heat the oven to 180°C/350°F/gas 4. Grease a 20 cm/8 inch square baking tin with olive oil spread.

Cut the sweet potatoes into small pieces and boil until just soft. Mash the potatoes, adding a little warm water to form a smooth mixture.

Meanwhile, sift the flours, cocoa powder and baking powder.

In a separate bowl, cream the olive oil spread with the sugar and vanilla essence then gradually mix in the eggs.

Add the dry ingredients, then mashed potato, and finally the chocolate. Pour the cake mix into the prepared tin and bake for 30 minutes.

This cake makes a lovely dessert served with cherries and a few spoonfuls of fromage frais or low fat Greek yoghurt.

Nutritional info per serving
1 fruit portion, 3 starchy food portions, 1 fat portion
230 kcal/961 kJ; Fat 10 g (monounsaturated 5 g, polyunsaturated 2 g, saturated 3 g); Protein 7 g; Carbohydrate 30 g; Fibre 2 g; Salt 0.5 g

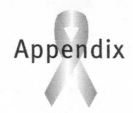

Appendix

Recording your progress

An important part of any weight loss plan is to monitor your progress, to check you are losing body fat. You should weigh yourself and take your waist and hip measurements once a week and record these measurements. (You can do this on the monitoring sheet opposite or photocopy it if you need more sheets.) You can use your weight and hip measurements to reassess your percentage body fat. I recommend that you do this every 2 weeks. (See the BMI Reckoner on page 266).

Tips for Monitoring Yourself
- Weight can fluctuate from day to day, so it is not a good idea to weigh yourself every day.
- Weight can change throughout the day, so always weigh and measure yourself at the same time of day – early in the morning is often easiest.
- Use the same set of reliable scales.
- Try to wear the same light clothing when you weigh yourself.
- Remember, some clothes may constrict your waist and hip measurements.
- Bear in mind that weight and waist measurements can often be bigger over the premenstrual days.

Goals			
	Body Fat	*Waist*	*Hips*
Starting point			
Goals			
My goals	To lose _____ of fat	To lose _____ off my waist	To lose _____ off my hips

Progress sheet					
Date	*Weight*	*Waist*	*Hips*	*Percentage body fat*	*Body fat lb/kg*

Food and exercise diary

Why keep a food and exercise diary?

- Keeping a record of what you eat and drink, when you eat and drink it and the amount of exercise you do will make you aware of your current diet and exercise habits.
- Seeing how well your current patterns of diet and exercise match the recommended level in the programme will give you pointers for further changes you can make that may help you to lose weight.
- Recording your diet and exercise level is a great way to reinforce any positive changes you are trying to make.
- You may want to use the diary to see what situations trigger you to eat or overeat.

How to fill in your food and exercise diary

- First, you will need to make lots of photocopies of the sample diary on the opposite page, as the aim is to fill it out at on least 4 days of the week, including a weekend day if possible.
- Write down everything you eat and drink the moment you eat it. Only record the food and drink actually eaten, rather than what is offered to you.
- Record portion sizes using household measures, e.g. 2 heaped tablespoons of cereals, 1 slice of bread.
- Remember to include all snacks you may have had including drinks.
- Record the time when the food or drink is eaten.
- Record how the food is cooked, e.g. fried, boiled, grilled, microwaved.
- Try to estimate the amount of butter/margarine eaten for the day.
- Try to estimate the amount of milk you have drunk over the course of the day.
- Write down any planned, organised exercise (i.e. aerobics), and any day-to-day activities (i.e. 15 minutes walking, half-hour gardening).

Date: ——————— Day: ———————

Food and drink record		
Time	*Food/Drink*	*Portion*
	Total volume milk	
	Total butter/margarine	

Activity record		
Time	*Activity*	*Duration*

Find Your BMI

To use the table, find your height in inches or metres in the left-hand column. Move across to your weight. The number at the top of the

BMI	19	20	21	22	23	24	25	26	27	28	29
Height in/m	Weight lb/kg										
58/1.47	91/41	96/44	100/45	105/48	110/50	115/52	119/54	124/56	129/58	134/61	138/63
59/1.50	94/43	99/45	104/47	109/49	114/52	119/54	124/56	128/58	133/60	138/63	143/65
60/1.52	97/44	102/46	107/49	112/51	118/54	123/56	128/58	133/60	138/63	143/65	148/67
61/1.55	100/45	106/48	111/50	116/53	122/55	127/58	132/60	137/62	143/65	148/67	153/69
62/1.57	104/47	109/49	115/52	120/54	57/126	131/59	136/62	142/64	147/67	153/69	158/72
63/1.60	107/49	113/51	118/54	124/56	130/59	135/61	141/64	146/66	152/69	158/72	163/74
64/1.62	110/50	116/53	122/55	128/58	134/61	140/64	145/66	151/68	157/71	163/74	169/77
65/1.65	114/52	120/54	126/57	132/60	138/63	144/65	150/68	156/71	162/74	168/76	174/79
66/1.68	118/54	124/56	130/59	136/62	142/64	148/67	155/70	161/73	167/76	173/78	179/81
67/1.70	121/55	127/58	134/61	140/64	146/66	153/69	159/72	166/75	172/78	178/81	185/84
68/1.72	125/57	131/59	138/63	144/65	151/68	158/72	164/74	171/78	177/80	184/84	190/86
69/1.75	128/58	135/61	142/64	149/68	155/70	162/74	169/77	176/80	182/83	189/86	196/89
70/1.78	132/60	139/63	146/66	153/69	160/73	167/76	174/79	181/82	188/85	195/88	202/92
71/1.80	136/62	143/65	150/68	157/71	165/75	172/78	179/81	186/84	193/88	200/91	208/94
72/1.83	140/64	147/67	154/70	162/74	169/77	177/80	184/84	191/87	199/90	206/94	213/97
73/1.85	144/65	151/68	159/72	166/75	174/79	182/83	189/86	197/89	204/93	212/96	219/99
74/1.88	148/67	155/70	163/74	171/78	179/81	186/84	194/88	202/92	210/95	218/99	225/102
75/1.90	152/69	160/73	168/76	176/80	184/84	192/87	200/91	208/94	216/98	224/102	232/105
76/1.93	156/71	164/74	172/78	180/82	189/86	197/89	205/93	213/97	221/100	230/104	238/108

column (in the shaded bar) is the body mass index (BMI) at that height and weight. Weights have been rounded off.

30	31	32	33	34	35	36	37	38	39	40
Weight lb/kg										
143/65	148/67	153/69	158/72	162/74	167/76	172/78	177/80	181/82	186/84	191/87
148/67	153/69	158/72	163/74	168/76	173/78	178/81	183/83	188/85	193/88	198/90
153/69	158/72	163/74	168/76	174/79	179/81	184/83	189/86	194/88	199/90	204/93
158/72	164/74	169/77	174/79	180/82	185/84	190/86	195/88	201/91	206/93	211/96
164/74	169/77	175/79	180/82	186/84	191/87	196/89	202/92	207/94	213/97	218/99
169/77	175/79	180/82	186/84	191/87	197/89	203/92	208/94	214/97	220/100	225/102
174/79	180/82	186/84	192/87	197/89	204/93	209/95	215/98	221/100	227/103	232/105
180/82	186/84	192/87	198/90	204/93	210/95	216/98	222/101	228/103	234/106	240/109
186/84	192/87	198/90	204/93	210/95	216/98	223/101	229/104	235/107	241/109	247/112
191/87	198/90	204/93	211/96	217/99	223/101	230/104	236/107	242/110	249/113	255/116
197/89	203/92	210/95	216/98	223/101	230/104	236/107	243/110	249/113	256/116	262/119
203/92	209/95	216/98	223/101	230/104	236/107	243/112	250/113	257/117	263/119	270/122
209/95	216/98	222/101	229/104	236/107	243/110	250/113	257/117	264/120	271/123	278/126
215/98	222/101	229/104	236/107	243/110	250/114	257/117	265/120	272/123	279/127	286/130
221/100	228/104	235/107	242/110	250/114	258/117	265/120	272/123	279/127	287/130	294/133
227/103	235/107	242/110	250/114	257/117	265/120	272/123	280/127	288/131	295/134	302/137
233/106	241/109	249/113	256/116	264/120	272/123	280/127	287/130	295/134	303/137	311/141
240/109	248/113	256/116	264/120	272/123	279/127	287/130	295/134	303/137	311/141	319/145
246/112	254/115	263/119	271/123	279/127	287/130	295/134	304/138	312/142	320/145	328/149

Notes

Part One

1. Ziegler RG, Hoover RN, Nomura AM, West DW, Wu AH, Pike MC *et al.* Relative weight, weight change, height, and breast cancer risk in Asian-American women. *J. Natl. Cancer Inst.* 1996;88:650-60.
2. Kosters JP, Gotzsche PC. Regular self-examination or clinical examination for early detection of breast cancer. *Cochrane Database Syst.Rev.* 2003;CD003373.
3. *7th Handbook on Cancer Prevention*, IARC, Lyons 2002. 2005.
4. Peto J, Collins N, Barfoot R, Seal S, Warren W, Rahman N *et al.* Prevalence of BRCA1 and BRCA2 gene mutations in patients with early-onset breast cancer. *J. Natl.Cancer Inst.* 1999;91:943-9.
5. Peto J, Mack TM. High constant incidence in twins and other relatives of women with breast cancer. *Nat.Genet.* 2000;26:411-4.
6. Claus EB, Risch N, Thompson WD. Genetic analysis of breast cancer in the cancer and steroid hormone study. *Am. J. Hum.Genet.* 1991;48:232-42.
7. Colditz GA, Willett WC, Hunter DJ, Stampfer MJ, Manson JE, Hennekens CH *et al.* Family history, age, and risk of breast cancer. Prospective data from the Nurses' Health Study. *JAMA* 1993;270:338-43.
8. Pharoah PD, Lipscombe JM, Redman KL, Day NE, Easton DF, Ponder BA. Familial predisposition to breast cancer in a British population: implications for prevention. *Eur. J. Cancer* 2000;36:773-9.
9. Nielsen M. Autopsy studies of the occurrence of cancerous, atypical and benign epithelial lesions in the female breast. *APMIS Suppl* 1989;10:1-56.
10. King MC, Marks JH, Mandell JB. Breast and ovarian cancer risks due to inherited mutations in BRCA1 and BRCA2. *Science* 2003;302:643-6.
11. Kowalska E, Narod SA, Huzarski T, Zajaczek S, Huzarska J, Gorski B *et al.* Increased rates of chromosome breakage in BRCA1 carriers are normalized by oral selenium supplementation. *Cancer Epidemiol.Biomarkers Prev.* 2005;14:1302-6.
12. Sellers TA, Kushi LH, Potter JD, Kaye SA, Nelson CL, McGovern PG *et al.* Effect of family history, body-fat distribution, and reproductive factors on the risk of postmenopausal breast cancer. *N.Engl.J. Med.* 1992;326:1323-9.
13. Zhang S, Hunter DJ, Forman MR, Rosner BA, Speizer FE, Colditz GA *et al.* Dietary carotenoids and vitamins A, C, and E and risk of breast cancer. *J. Natl.Cancer Inst.* 1999;91:547-56.
14. Eaton SB, Pike MC, Short RV, Lee NC, Trussell J, Hatcher RA *et al.* Women's reproductive cancers in evolutionary context. *Q.Rev.Biol.* 1994;69:353-67.
15. Cauley JA, Gutai JP, Kuller LH, LeDonne D, Powell JG. The epidemiology of serum sex hormones in postmenopausal women. *Am. J. Epidemiol.* 1989;129:1120-31.
16. Rossouw JE, Anderson GL, Prentice RL, LaCroix AZ, Kooperberg C, Stefanick ML *et al.* Risks and benefits of estrogen plus progestin in healthy postmenopausal women: principal results from the Women's Health Initiative randomized controlled trial. *JAMA* 2002;288:321-33.
17. Beral V. Breast cancer and hormone-replacement therapy in the Million Women Study. *Lancet* 2003;362:419-27.
18. Wolff MS, Toniolo PG, Lee EW, Rivera M, Dubin N. Blood levels of organochlorine residues and risk of breast cancer. *J. Natl.Cancer Inst.* 1993;85:648-52.
19. Coyle YM. The effect of environment on breast cancer risk. *Breast Cancer Res.Treat.* 2004;84:273-88.
20. Gammon MD, Santella RM, Neugut AI, Eng SM, Teitelbaum SL, Paykin A *et al.* Environmental toxins and breast cancer on Long Island. I. Polycyclic aromatic hydrocarbon DNA adducts. *Cancer Epidemiol.Biomarkers Prev.* 2002;11:677-85.

Notes

21. Aschengrau A, Coogan PF, Quinn M, Cashins LJ. Occupational exposure to estrogenic chemicals and the occurrence of breast cancer: an exploratory analysis. *Am. J. Ind.Med.* 1998;34:6-14.
22. Golden R, Gandy J, Vollmer G. A review of the endocrine activity of parabens and implications for potential risks to human health. *Crit. Rev.Toxicol.* 2005;35:435-58.
23. Atkinson D, Burnett F, Foster G N, Litterick A, Mullay M and C A. The minimisation of pesticide residues of food a review of the published literature. 2005.
    Ref Type: Generic
24. Soil Association. *Soil Association Organic farming, food quality and health. A review of the evidence.* 2001. Bristol.
25. Gram IT, Braaten T, Terry PD, Sasco AJ, Adami HO, Lund E *et al.* Breast cancer risk among women who start smoking as teenagers. *Cancer Epidemiol.Biomarkers Prev.* 2005;14:61-6.
26. Zheng W, Deitz AC, Campbell DR, Wen WQ, Cerhan JR, Sellers TA *et al.* N-acetyltransferase 1 genetic polymorphism, cigarette smoking, well-done meat intake, and breast cancer risk. *Cancer Epidemiol.Biomarkers Prev.* 1999;8:233-9.
27. Nielsen NR, Zhang ZF, Kristensen TS, Netterstrom B, Schnohr P, Gronbaek M. Self reported stress and risk of breast cancer: prospective cohort study. *BMJ* 2005;331:548.
28. Graham J, Ramirez A, Love S, Richards M, Burgess C. Stressful life experiences and risk of relapse of breast cancer: observational cohort study. *BMJ* 2002;324:1420.

Part Two

1. Matkovic V, Ilich JZ, Skugor M, Badenhop NE, Goel P, Clairmont A *et al.* Leptin is inversely related to age at menarche in human females. *J. Clin. Endocrinol. Metab.* 1997;82:3239-45.
2. van den Brandt PA, Spiegelman D, Yaun SS, Adami HO, Beeson L, Folsom AR *et al.* Pooled analysis of prospective cohort studies on height, weight, and breast cancer risk. *Am. J. Epidemiol.* 2000;152:514-27.
3. Tretli S, Gaard M. Lifestyle changes during adolescence and risk of breast cancer: an ecologic study of the effect of World War II in Norway. *Cancer Causes Control* 1996;7:507-12.
4. Huang Z, Hankinson SE, Colditz GA, Stampfer MJ, Hunter DJ, Manson JE *et al.* Dual effects of weight and weight gain on breast cancer risk. *JAMA* 1997;278:1407-11.
5. Harvie M, Howell A, Vierkant RA, Kumar N, Cerhan JR, Kelemen LE *et al.* Association of gain and loss of weight before and after menopause with risk of postmenopausal breast cancer in the Iowa women's health study. *Cancer Epidemiol.Biomarkers Prev.* 2005;14:656-61.
6. Lahmann PH, Lissner L, Gullberg B, Olsson H, Berglund G. A prospective study of adiposity and postmenopausal breast cancer risk: the Malmö Diet and Cancer Study. *Int.J. Cancer* 2003;103:246-52.
7. Harvie M, Hooper L, Howell AH. Central obesity and breast cancer risk: a systematic review. *Obes.Rev.* 2003;4:157-73.
8. Silvera SA, Jain M, Howe GR, Miller AB, Rohan TE. Energy balance and breast cancer risk: a prospective cohort study. *Breast Cancer Res.Treat.* 2005;1-10.
9. Harvie M, Mercer T, Alford D, Malik R, Adams J, and Howell A. The effect of weight loss and weight gain on biomarkers of breast cancer risk. Cancer Epidemiol.Biomarkers Prev. Proceedings of American Association of Cancer Research 2nd Frontiers in Cancer Prevention Conference (12), 11. 2003.
10. Naimi TS, Brown DW, Brewer RD, Giles WH, Mensah G, Serdula MK *et al.* Cardiovascular risk factors and confounders among nondrinking and moderate-drinking U.S. adults. *Am. J. Prev.Med.* 2005;28:369-73.
11. Rohan TE, Jain MG, Howe GR, Miller AB. Dietary folate consumption and breast cancer risk. *J. Natl.Cancer Inst.* 2000;92:266-9.

12. Zhang S, Hunter DJ, Hankinson SE, Giovannucci EL, Rosner BA, Colditz GA et al. A prospective study of folate intake and the risk of breast cancer. JAMA 1999;281:1632-7.

13. Baglietto L, English DR, Gertig DM, Hopper JL, Giles GG. Does dietary folate intake modify effect of alcohol consumption on breast cancer risk? Prospective cohort study. BMJ 2005;331:807.

14. Baker JA, Beehler GP, Sawant AC, Jayaprakash V, McCann SE, Moysich KB. Consumption of coffee, but not black tea, is associated with decreased risk of premenopausal breast cancer. J. Nutr. 2006;136:166-71.

15. Nkondjock A, Ghadirian P, Kotsopoulos J, Lubinski J, Lynch H, Kim-Sing C et al. Coffee consumption and breast cancer risk among BRCA1 and BRCA2 mutation carriers. Int. J. Cancer 2006;118:103-7.

16. Chobanian AV, Bakris GL, Black HR, Cushman WC, Green LA, Izzo JL Jr. et al. Seventh report of the Joint National Committee on Prevention, Detection, Evaluation, and Treatment of High Blood Pressure. Hypertension 2003;42:1206-52.

17. Nawrot P, Jordan S, Eastwood J, Rotstein J, Hugenholtz A, Feeley M. Effects of caffeine on human health. Food Addit.Contam. 2003;20:1-30.

18. Sun CL, Yuan JM, Koh WP, Yu MC. Green tea, black tea and breast cancer risk: a meta-analysis of epidemiological studies. Carcinogenesis 2005.

19. Geleijnse JM, Launer LJ, Van der Kuip DA, Hofman A, Witteman JC. Inverse association of tea and flavonoid intakes with incident myocardial infarction: the Rotterdam Study. Am. J. Clin. Nutr. 2002;75:880-6.

20. Bingham SA, Luben R, Welch A, Wareham N, Khaw KT, Day N. Are imprecise methods obscuring a relation between fat and breast cancer? Lancet 2003;362:212–14.

21. Voorrips LE, Brants HA, Kardinaal AF, Hiddink GJ, van den Brandt PA, Goldbohm RA. Intake of conjugated linoleic acid, fat, and other fatty acids in relation to postmenopausal breast cancer: the Netherlands Cohort Study on Diet and Cancer. Am. J. Clin. Nutr. 2002;76:873-82.

22. The World Health Organisation global strategy for diet physical activity and health. 2005. http://www.who.int/gb/ebwha/pdf_files/WHA57/A57_R17-en.pdf

23. Smith-Warner SA, Spiegelman D, Yaun SS, Adami HO, Beeson WL, van den Brandt PA et al. Intake of fruits and vegetables and risk of breast cancer: a pooled analysis of cohort studies. JAMA 2001;285:769-76.

24. van Gils CH, Peeters PH, Bueno-de-Mesquita HB, Boshuizen HC, Lahmann PH, Clavel-Chapelon F et al. Consumption of vegetables and fruits and risk of breast cancer. JAMA 2005;293:183-93.

25. Terry P, Wolk A, Persson I, Magnusson C. Brassica vegetables and breast cancer risk. JAMA 2001;285:2975-7.

26. Sato R, Helzlsouer KJ, Alberg AJ, Hoffman SC, Norkus EP, Comstock GW. Prospective study of carotenoids, tocopherols, and retinoid concentrations and the risk of breast cancer. Cancer Epidemiol.Biomarkers Prev. 2002;11:451-7.

27. Dorgan JF, Sowell A, Swanson CA, Potischman N, Miller R, Schussler N et al. Relationships of serum carotenoids, retinol, alpha-tocopherol, and selenium with breast cancer risk: results from a prospective study in Columbia, Missouri (United States). Cancer Causes Control 1998;9:89-97.

28. Toniolo P, Van Kappel AL, Akhmedkhanov A, Ferrari P, Kato I, Shore RE et al. Serum carotenoids and breast cancer. Am. J. Epidemiol. 2001;153:1142-7.

29. Zhang S, Hunter DJ, Forman MR, Rosner BA, Speizer FE, Colditz GA et al. Dietary carotenoids and vitamins A, C, and E and risk of breast cancer. J. Natl.Cancer Inst. 1999;91:547-56.

30. Khaw KT, Bingham S, Welch A, Luben R, Wareham N, Oakes S et al. Relation between plasma ascorbic acid and mortality in men and women in EPIC-Norfolk prospective study: a prospective population study. European Prospective Investigation into Cancer and Nutrition. Lancet 2001;357:657-63.

31. Olsen A, Knudsen KE, Thomsen BL, Loft S, Stripp C, Overvad K et al. Plasma enterolactone and breast cancer incidence by estrogen receptor status. Cancer Epidemiol.Biomarkers Prev. 2004;13:2084-9.

32. Adebamowo CA, Cho E, Sampson L, Katan MB, Spiegelman D, Willett WC et al. Dietary flavonols and flavonol-rich foods intake and the risk of breast cancer. *Int. J. Cancer* 2005;114:628-33.

33. Conaway CC, Getahun SM, Liebes LL, Pusateri DJ, Topham DK, Botero-Omary M et al. Disposition of glucosinolates and sulforaphane in humans after ingestion of steamed and fresh broccoli. *Nutr.Cancer* 2000;38:168-78.

34. Verkerk R, Dekker M. Glucosinolates and myrosinase activity in red cabbage (Brassica oleracea L. var. Capitata f. rubra DC.) after various microwave treatments. *J. Agric.Food Chem.* 2004;52:7318-23.

35. Donovan SM, Chao JC, Zijlstra RT, Odle J. Orally administered iodinated recombinant human insulin-like growth factor-I (125I-rhIGF-I) is poorly absorbed by the newborn piglet. *J. Pediatr.Gastroenterol.Nutr.* 1997;24:174-82.

36. Moorman PG, Terry PD. Consumption of dairy products and the risk of breast cancer: a review of the literature. *Am. J. Clin. Nutr.* 2004;80:5-14.

37. Shin MH, Holmes MD, Hankinson SE, Wu K, Colditz GA, Willett WC. Intake of dairy products, calcium, and vitamin D and risk of breast cancer. *J. Natl.Cancer Inst.* 2002;94:1301-11.

38. Ibid.

39. McCullough ML, Rodriguez C, Diver WR, Feigelson HS, Stevens VL, Thun MJ. et al. Dairy, calcium, and vitamin D intake and postmenopausal breast cancer risk in the Cancer Prevention Study II Nutrition Cohort. *Cancer Epidemiol.Biomarkers Prev.* 2005;14:2898-904.

40. Cho E, Smith-Warner SA, Spiegelman D, Beeson WL, van den Brandt PA, Colditz GA et al. Dairy foods, calcium, and colorectal cancer: a pooled analysis of 10 cohort studies. *J. Natl.Cancer Inst.* 2004;96:1015-22.

41. Ip MM, Masso-Welch PA, Ip C. Prevention of mammary cancer with conjugated linoleic acid: role of the stroma and the epithelium. *J. Mammary. Gland. Biol. Neoplasia.* 2003;8:103-18.

42. Slavin J. Why whole grains are protective: biological mechanisms. *Proc.Nutr.Soc.* 2003;62:129-34.

43. Rose DP, Lubin M, Connolly JM. Effects of diet supplementation with wheat bran on serum estrogen levels in the follicular and luteal phases of the menstrual cycle. *Nutrition* 1997;13:535-9.

44. Silvera SA, Jain M, Howe GR, Miller AB, Rohan TE. Dietary carbohydrates and breast cancer risk: a prospective study of the roles of overall glycemic index and glycemic load. *Int. J. Cancer* 2005;114:653-8.

45. Cho E, Spiegelman D, Hunter DJ, Chen WY, Colditz GA, Willett WC. Premenopausal dietary carbohydrate, glycemic index, glycemic load, and fiber in relation to risk of breast cancer. *Cancer Epidemiol.Biomarkers Prev.* 2003;12:1153-8.

46. Clifton P. Wholegrain is better than other heart heath foods despite high GI. 2005. http://www.medicalnewstoday.com/medicalnews.php?newsid=25073

47. Gago-Dominguez M, Yuan JM, Sun CL, Lee HP, Yu MC. Opposing effects of dietary n-3 and n-6 fatty acids on mammary carcinogenesis: The Singapore Chinese Health Study. *Br.J. Cancer* 2003;89:1686-92.

48. Advice on fish consumption benefits and risk. 2005. http://www.food.gov.uk/multimedia/pdfs/fishreport2004full.pdf

49. Zheng W, Deitz AC, Campbell DR, Wen WQ, Cerhan JR, Sellers TA et al. N-acetyltransferase 1 genetic polymorphism, cigarette smoking, well-done meat intake, and breast cancer risk. *Cancer Epidemiol.Biomarkers Prev.* 1999;8:233-9.

50. Mucci LA, Sandin S, Balter K, Adami HO, Magnusson C, Weiderpass E. Acrylamide intake and breast cancer risk in Swedish women. *JAMA* 2005;293:1326-7.

51. Weihrauch MR, Diehl V. Artificial sweeteners—do they bear a carcinogenic risk? *Ann.Oncol.* 2004; 15:1460-5.

52. Hunter DJ, Manson JE, Colditz GA, Stampfer MJ, Rosner B, Hennekens CH et al. A prospective study of the intake of vitamins C, E, and A and the risk of breast cancer. *N. Engl. J. Med.* 1993;329:234-40.

53. Hercberg S, Galan P, Preziosi P, Bertrais S, Mennen L, Malvy D et al. The SU.VI.MAX Study: a randomized, placebo-controlled trial of the health effects of antioxidant vitamins and minerals. Arch.Intern.Med. 2004;164:2335-42.

54. Caraballoso M, Sacristan M, Serra C, Bonfill X. Drugs for preventing lung cancer in healthy people. Cochrane Database Syst. Rev. 2003;CD002141.

55. Bjelakovic G, Nikolova D, Simonetti RG, Gluud C. Antioxidant supplements for preventing gastrointestinal cancers. Cochrane Database Syst. Rev. 2004;CD004183.

56. Expert group on vitamins and minerals. Safe upper limits for vitamins and minerals. 2005. London, Food Standard Agency. Ref Type: Generic.

57. Lamartiniere CA. Timing of exposure and mammary cancer risk. J. Mammary Gland Biol. Neoplasia. 2002;7:67-76.

58. Shu XO, Jin F, Dai Q, Wen W, Potter JD, Kushi LH et al. Soyfood intake during adolescence and subsequent risk of breast cancer among Chinese women. Cancer Epidemiol, Biomarkers Prev. 2001;10:483-8.

59. The Committee on Toxicity of chemicals in food / consumer products and the environment Phytoestrogens and Health. 2003. London, Food Standards Agency. Ref Type: Generic.

60. Hargreaves DF, Potten CS, Harding C, Shaw LE, Morton MS, Roberts SA et al. Two-week dietary soy supplementation has an estrogenic effect on normal premenopausal breast. J. Clin. Endocrinol. Metab. 1999;84:4017-24.

61. Petrakis NL, Barnes S, King EB, Lowenstein J, Wiencke J, Lee MM et al. Stimulatory influence of soy protein isolate on breast secretion in pre- and postmenopausal women. Cancer Epidemiol.Biomarkers Prev. 1996;5:785-94.

62. Grace PB, Taylor JI, Low YL, Luben RN, Mulligan AA, Botting NP et al. Phytoestrogen concentrations in serum and spot urine as biomarkers for dietary phytoestrogen intake and their relation to breast cancer risk in European prospective investigation of cancer and nutrition-Norfolk. Cancer Epidemiol.Biomarkers Prev. 2004;13:698-708.

63. Atkinson C, Warren RM, Sala E, Dowsett M, Dunning AM, Healey CS et al. Red-clover-derived isoflavones and mammographic breast density: a double-blind, randomized, placebo-controlled trial [ISRCTN42940165]. Breast Cancer Res. 2004; 6:R170-R179.

64. Thune I, Furberg AS. Physical activity and cancer risk: dose-response and cancer, all sites and site-specific. Med.Sci.Sports Exerc. 2001;33:S530-S550.

65. Lagerros YT, Hsieh SF, Hsieh CC. Physical activity in adolescence and young adulthood and breast cancer risk: a quantitative review. Eur. J. Cancer Prev. 2004;13:5-12.

66. McTiernan A, Ulrich CM, Yancey D, Slate S, Nakamura H, Oestreicher N et al. The Physical Activity for Total Health (PATH) Study: rationale and design. Med.Sci.Sports Exerc. 1999;31:1307-12.

67. Harvie MN, Campbell IT, Baildam A, Howell A. Energy balance in early breast cancer patients receiving adjuvant chemotherapy. Breast Cancer Res.Treat. 2004;83:201-10.

68. Kroenke CH, Chen WY, Rosner B, Holmes MD. Weight, weight gain, and survival after breast cancer diagnosis. J. Clin. Oncol. 2005;23:1370-8.

69. Dignam JJ, Wieand K, Johnson KA, Fisher B, Xu L, Mamounas EP. Obesity, tamoxifen use, and outcomes in women with estrogen receptor-positive early-stage breast cancer. J. Natl.Cancer Inst. 2003;95:1467-76.

70. Harvie M, Howell A. The need for lifestyle interventions amongst post menopausal women with early breast cancer. Women's Health 2005;1(2):205-23. 9-9-0005.

71. Turner LE, McDowell G, Parker R and Bundred NJ. Does flaxseed relieve vasomotor symptoms? Breast Cancer Res. 88 (suppl. 1), 239.12-12-0004.

Part Three

1. Peeters A, Barendregt JJ, Willekens F, Mackenbach JP, Al Mamun A, Bonneux L. Obesity in adulthood and its consequences for life expectancy: a life-table analysis. Ann. Intern. Med. 2003;138:24-32.

2. Weigle DS, Breen PA, Matthys CC, Callahan HS, Meeuws KE, Burden VR *et al.* A high-protein diet induces sustained reductions in appetite, ad libitum caloric intake, and body weight despite compensatory changes in diurnal plasma leptin and ghrelin concentrations. *Am. J. Clin. Nutr.* 2005;82:41-8.

3. Jacobsen R, Lorenzen JK, Toubro S, Krog-Mikkelsen I, Astrup A. Effect of short-term high dietary calcium intake on 24-h energy expenditure, fat oxidation, and fecal fat excretion. *Int. J. Obes.(Lond.)* 2005;29:292-301.

4. Liu S, Willett WC, Manson JE, Hu FB, Rosner B, Colditz G. Relation between changes in intakes of dietary fiber and grain products and changes in weight and development of obesity among middle-aged women. *Am. J. Clin. Nutr.* 2003;78:920-7.

5. Farshchi HR, Taylor MA, Macdonald IA. Beneficial metabolic effects of regular meal frequency on dietary thermogenesis, insulin sensitivity, and fasting lipid profiles in healthy obese women. *Am. J. Clin. Nutr.* 2005;81:16-24.

6. Farshchi HR, Taylor MA, Macdonald IA. Deleterious effects of omitting breakfast on insulin sensitivity and fasting lipid profiles in healthy lean women. *Am. J. Clin. Nutr.* 2005;81:388-96.

7. Wing RR, Phelan S. Long-term weight loss maintenance. *Am. J. Clin. Nutr.* 2005;82:222S-5S.

8. Wing RR, Jeffery RW. Prescribed "breaks" as a means to disrupt weight control efforts. *Obes.Res.* 2003;11:287-91.

9. Bertone-Johnson ER, Hankinson SE, Bendich A, Johnson SR, Willett WC, Manson JE. Calcium and vitamin D intake and risk of incident premenstrual syndrome. *Arch.Intern.Med.* 2005;165:1246-52.

Resources

UK

Information and Support

Breast Cancer Care
www.breastcancercare.org.uk
Kiln House
210 New Kings Road
London SW6 4NZ
Tel: 0808 800 6000
Email: info@breastcancercare.org.uk
Breast Cancer Care is the UK's leading charity for breast cancer information
and support.

CancerBACUP
www.CancerBACUP.org.uk
3 Bath Place
Rivington Street
London EC2 3JR
Tel: 020 7696 9003
CancerBACUP is a UK charity providing information, as
well as emotional support and counselling to people living
with cancer.

Lavender Trust
www.breastcancercare.org.uk/content.php?page_id=512
Advice and information for young women diagnosed with breast cancer.

The Cancer Counselling Trust
www.cctrust.org.uk
1 Noel Road
London N1 8HQ
Tel: 020 7704 1137
Email: support@cctrust.org.uk
In-person and telephone counselling for cancer patients, their families,
friends and care givers.

Cancer Research

Breast Cancer Campaign
www.bcc-uk.org
Clifton Centre
110 Clifton Street
London EC2A 4HT
Tel: 020 7749 3700
Breast Cancer Campaign funds research into breast cancer. Their website
offers a range of information on the disease.

Cancer Research UK
www.cancerresearchuk.org
PO Box 123
Lincoln's Inn Fields
London WC2A 3PX
Tel: 020 7242 0200
Dedicated to research on the causes, treatment and prevention of cancer.

The Genesis Appeal
www.genesisuk.org
PO Box 320
Manchester M20 2HT
Tel: 08700 62 3000
The Genesis Appeal supports vital research into breast cancer prevention and in 2007 will open Europe's first purpose-built breast cancer prevention centre.

World Cancer Research Fund
www.wcrf-uk.org
19 Harley Street
London W1G 9QL
Tel: 020 7343 4200
Information on cancer prevention, including booklets that can be downloaded from the web, for the general public and health professionals.

Diet and Nutrition

British Dietetic Association
www.bda.uk.com
5th Floor
Charles House
148/9 Great Charles Street
Queensway
Birmingham B3 3HT
Tel: 0121 200 8080
Email: info@bda.uk.com
Advice on finding a dietician or other nutrition expert.

British Nutrition Foundation
www.nutrition.org.uk
High Holborn House
Holborn
London WC1 6RQ
Tel: 020 7404 6747
Email: postbox@nutrition.org.uk
A useful source of information covering all aspects of food and diet.

National Obesity Forum
www.nationalobesityforum.org.uk
PO Box 6625
Nottingham NG2 5PA
Tel: 0115 846 2109
Email: info@nationalobesityforum.org.uk
A valuable source of information plus good links and research.

Weight Concern
www.weightconcern.org.uk
Brook House
2–16 Torrington Place
London WC1E 7HN
Tel: 020 7679 6636
Email: enquiries@weightconcern.org.uk
This registered charity, dedicated to fighting the UK's obesity epidemic, has a very useful website.

Other Useful Sources of Information

Bristol Cancer Help Centre
www.bristolcancerhelp.org.uk
Tel: 0845 123 23 10
The UK's leading holistic cancer charity.

British Columbia Cancer Agency
www.bccancer.bc.ca
Good information on cancer, including advice on prevention.

British Heart Foundation National Centre for Physical Activity and Health
www.bhfactive.org.uk/links
A great source of links to exercise, fitness and health information.

Cancer risk prediction
www.yourdiseaserisk.harvard.edu
A cancer risk assessment tool devised by the Harvard Center for Cancer Prevention.

Cancer screening
www.cancerscreening.nhs.uk
Information on the NHS screening programme; also provides publications about breast screening.

Giving up smoking
Quit
www.quit.org.uk
Tel: 0800 00 22 00
Help and advice for people who want to give up smoking.

Memorial Sloane Kettering Cancer Centre
www.mskcc.org
Information on cancer for patients and professionals.

National Hereditary Breast Cancer Helpline
Tel: 01629 813 000
Advice on genetic testing and prophylactic surgery.

National Osteoporosis Society
www.nos.org.uk
Information on osteoporosis, and advice on prevention and treatment. The website includes a quiz to assess your risk of developing the condition.

Australia

The National Breast Cancer Centre (NBCC)
www.nbcc.org.au
92 Parramatta Road
Camperdown NSW 2050
Australia
Tel: 2 9036 3030
Email: directorate@nbcc.org.au
The NBCC provides information, resources and programmes for women with breast cancer, the media, health care professionals and the general public.

Breast Health (part of the NBCC)
www.breasthealth.com.au
Information and advice on breast health for all women, whether they have been diagnosed with breast cancer or are concerned about staying healthy.

The Breast Cancer Network Australia
www.bcna.org.au
293 Camberwell Rd
Camberwell VIC 3124
Australia
Tel: 3 9805 2500
Email: beacon@bcna.org.au
Information and support for people whose lives have been affected by breast cancer, including a range of kits for women who have just been diagnosed with the disease.

The National Breast Cancer Foundation
www.nbcf.org.au
GPO Box 4126
Sydney NSW 2001
Tel: 2 9299 4090
Email: info@nbcf.org.au
This organisation raises funds to support all forms of research into breast cancer prevention and the search for a cure.

Nutrition Australia
www.nutritionaustralia.org
Information on food and healthy eating.

Quit
www.quit.org.au
Tel: 13 78 48
Help and advice for people who want to stop smoking.

New Zealand

The New Zealand Breast Cancer Foundation
www.nzbcf.org.nz
PO Box 99 650
Newmarket, Auckland
Tel: 09 523 4397
Information on breast cancer, including advice on useful resources for people with the disease. The Foundation aims to reduce the number of cases of breast cancer in New Zealand, and improve outcomes for those who are diagnosed with the disease.

The Cancer Society of New Zealand
www.cancernz.org.nz
PO Box 10847
Wellington 6036
Tel: 04 494 7270
Information and advice on the prevention and treatment of all types of cancer, as well as support for those whose lives have been affected by cancer.

EveryBody
www.everybody.co.nz
Information on a range of health issues including nutrition and breast cancer.

Quit
www.quit.co.nz
PO Box 12605
Wellington
Tel: 0800 778 778
Support and advice for people who want to stop smoking.

South Africa

Breast Cancer South Africa
www.breastcancer.co.za
Information on breast cancer and specialist clinics in South Africa.

The Cancer Association of South Africa (CANSA)
www.cansa.org.za
PO Box 2121
Bedfordview
Johannesburg 2008
Gauteng South Africa
Tel: 0800 226 622
CANSA provides information and support to people whose lives have been affected by cancer, as well as support for research into the disease.

Breast Care Centre for Excellence and the Breast Care Foundation
www.breasthealth.co.za
Tel: 0860 233 233
Email: breasthealth@netcare.co.za
Information on the treatment of breast health problems, including breast cancer.

South African Health Information
www.sahealthinfo.org
Information on a range of health issues, including nutrition and cancer.

Recipe Index

Index

National Surgical Adjuvant Breast and Bowel Project 143
National Toxicology Programme Report 45
National Weight Control Registry, USA 186
natural remedies 143–5, **146–7**
neotame 106
New Zealand 19, 20, 29, 64, 94–5, 109, 111, 153
Nielsen, Maya 33
nitrosamines 102
Norway 64
Nurses' Health Study, USA 78, 90, 95, 148, 173, 187
nuts 85, 92, 116, 172, 173
Brazil nuts 109, 116, 173

Obesity Reviews 71
oesophagus, cancer of 87, 107
oestradiol 37
oestrogen 25, 45, 49, 80, 89, 94, 112, 126
in HRT 40–1, 66–7
promotes cancer 26–7, 35–6, 37–8, 70, 71, 75, 97, 113, 138
Ohio State University 64
oils, olive/vegetable 85
omega-3 fats 83, 85–6, 92, 101, 116, 140, 180
omega-6 fats 83, 85–6, 101
oral contraceptives 39, 44
organic food 48–9
Orlistat (Xenical Roche) 160
osteoporosis 41–2, 104, 111, 117, 126, 148
Oxford University 39

PAHs (polycyclic aromatic hydro-carbons) 45, 102
pain, breast 29
pancreatic cancer 107
parabens 45, 47
Pauling, Linus 108
PCBs (polychlorinated biphenyls) 44–5, 45–6, 101–2
PCHs (polycyclic hydrocarbons) 46–7
periods 25, 29, 37, 125–6
see also menarche; menopause
pesticides 45–7, 50
Peto, Professor Julian 32
phthalates 47
Physical Activity and Total Health Study, Seattle 126
phytochemicals 87
phytoestrogens 91, 115

polyphenols 78, 81, 90–1, 97
poultry 85, 101–3, 172
pregnancy 43, 44, 159, 167
premenstrual syndrome 187
Prentice, Professor 177
processed foods 103–5, **105**, 174
procyanids 91
Professor Narod Centre for Research in Women's Health, Toronto 80
progesterone 25, 27, 37, 71, 75, 94
in HRT 40–1
progesterone-only contraceptives 39
prolactin 37
protein foods
healthy diet quiz 118–19, 121
and weight loss **169**, 171–2
pulses and beans 91–2
healthy diet quiz 118, 120

quercetin 91

radiation 47
radiotherapy 130, 138, 148–9
ready reckoners
body fat 68–9, **72–3**
healthy diet quiz 118–123
reproductive factors in breast cancer risk 37–8, **44**
resveratrol 91, 92
risk factors of breast cancer 57
Rowe, Silvena 195
Royal Marsden Hospital, London 149
Royal Veterinary and Agricultural University, Denmark 172

saccharin 106
SAD (seasonal affective disorder) 187–8
salt 103–5, **105**
healthy diet quiz 120, 123
Second World War 64
selenium 26, 36, 92, 97, 107, 108, **109**, 116
selenium methionine 108, 109
Sellers, Professor Tom 66
serotonin 187–8
Shanghai Breast Cancer Study 113–4
Shaw, Dr Clare 149
Sibutramine (Reductil, Abbott) 160
skin cancer 95–6
sleep deprivation 188
smoking 48, 159
snacks
healthy snack foods 179–80
serving sizes for weight loss **171**
snack meals 177

Genesis

creating a future without breast cancer

Please help to play a part in fighting this disease. You could become a Friend of Genesis or receive further details on the charity. Simply complete the following form, detach and send to:

The Genesis Appeal
PO Box 320
Manchester
M20 2HT

☐ I wish to make a donation to the Genesis Appeal and help the
fight against Breast Cancer.   £...............

☐ I wish to become a Friend of Genesis for £10.00 a year   £...............

☐ I would like more information on the Genesis Appeal

Name: _____

Address: _____

_____

Post Code: _____ Tel No: _____

Please make all cheques payable to **The Genesis Appeal**

If you wish to make your donation by Mastercard/Visa/Maestro (delete as applicable)
please fill in your details below.

Issue Number (Maestro Only): _ _

Card No: _ _ _ _   _ _ _ _   _ _ _ _   _ _ _ _

Start Date: _ _ /_ _   Expiry: _ _ /_ _

Signed: _____ Total: £ ....

Security Code: _ _ _ *Please supply the last 3 digits from the number on the reverse
of your card*

gift aid it

Using Gift Aid means that for every pound you give, we get an extra 28 pence from
the Inland Revenue, helping your donation go further. This means that £10.00 can be
turned into £12.80, just so long as the donations are made through Gift Aid. Imagine
what a difference that could make and it doesn't cost you a thing. So if you want your
donation to go further, Gift Aid it. Just tick this box and return the form.

I want all donations I've made since 6 April 2000 and all donations in the future to be
Gift Aid until I notify you otherwise. ☐

To qualify for Gift Aid, what you pay in income tax or capital gains tax must at least
equal the amount we will claim in the tax year.

Registered Charity No. 1109839